17·37

369 0229916

KU-331-968

History Taking
in Medicine and Surgery

Third Edition

M. Fishman

BM BCh (Oxon.), MA (Cantab.), BA (Hons.) M   S Eng.), PhD
G   Cambridge
                                          al Schools

M. Cullen

MB BS   C. (Hons.), nMRCGP, DFSRH
Graduate of Imperial College, London

Edited by **Ashley Grossman**

FmedSci
BA, BSc, MD, FRCP
Professor of Endocrinology
University of Oxford

Dedicated to your success

© 2014 PASTEST LTD
Egerton Court
Parkgate Estate
Knutsford
Cheshire
WA16 8DX
Telephone: 01565 752000

First Published 2005
Second Edition 2010
Third Edition 2014

ISBN: 1 905635 91 5
ISBN: 978 1 905635 91 7

A catalogue record for this book is available from the British Library. The information contained within this book was obtained by the authors from reliable sources. However, while every effort has been made to ensure its accuracy, no responsibility for loss, damage or injury occasioned to any person acting or refraining from action as a result of information contained herein can be accepted by the publishers or authors.

PasTest Revision Books and Intensive Courses
PasTest has been established in the field of postgraduate medical education since 1972, providing revision books and intensive study courses for doctors preparing for their professional examinations.

Books and courses are available for the following specialties:

MRCGP, MRCP Parts 1 and 2, MRCPCH Parts 1 and 2, MRCS, MRCOG, PLAB Parts 1 and 2 Dental Students and Dentists.
For further details contact:

PasTest, Freepost, Knutsford, Cheshire WA16 7BR
Tel: 01565 752000   **Fax: 01565 650264**
www.pastest.co.uk   **enquires@pastest.co.uk**

Text prepared by Carnegie Book Production, Lancaster.
Printed and bound in the UK by CPI Antony Rowe

Contents

Foreword to the third edition

It is rare nowadays for any book to achieve a 3rd edition, and when it occurs it usually signifies a text of great value, considerable utility, or both. I am therefore really pleased to endorse this new edition of Jonathan and Laura Fishman's *History Taking in Medicine and Surgery*, which has now proven itself as an informative and useful guide to clinical history taking in both medicine and surgery. I have emphasised in previous Forewords how important classic history taking is in clinical medicine, even, or may be especially, when there is now such a plethora of different sources of patient information, from blood and urine investigations, radiological studies including the most recent functional PET imaging, and even molecular biological '–omics' studies using DNA, RNA, protein or metabolomic arrays. All are being increasingly designed to personalise medical care and therapy, but the most personal of all is a careful and precise clinical history. Indeed, there is little point in any of this 'customisation' if there is inaccurate diagnosis, and the essence of this remains a competent clinical history and associated examination. This remains the cornerstone of clinical medicine, from which all else flows.

Clinical history taking should be fun: it is like reading a good detective story, clues abound, and the prize for being right is not only a feeling of satisfaction, but more importantly establishing the correct diagnosis optimises the patient's subsequent management; this is true 'personalised medicine'.

This edition has been updated with more and newer case studies. It will of course be extremely helpful for young physicians taking both basic and higher examinations, but at the same time I am sure that aspiring as well as established doctors will find it enthusing and enjoyable.

Ashley Grossman FmedSci

Professor of Endocrinology
Churchill Hospital
University of Oxford

About the authors

Jonathan M. Fishman BA (Hons), MA (Cantab), BM BCh (Oxon), MRCS (Eng), DOHNS (RCS Eng), PhD

Jonathan is a Specialist Registrar in ENT and a member of the Royal College of Surgeons. He graduated with a triple first class honours degree in Natural Sciences from Sidney Sussex College, University of Cambridge and completed his clinical training at St John's College, Oxford and the John Radcliffe Hospital. Jonathan spent part of his medical training at both Harvard University and NASA space centre.

Jonathan has extensive teaching experience and is primary author of six undergraduate and postgraduate medical textbooks. Jonathan was awarded Taylor and Howard-Agg Scholarships at Sidney Sussex College, Cambridge and has been awarded the highly prestigious title of "Lifelong Honorary Scholar", by the University of Cambridge, for academic excellence. In 2009 he was awarded the Royal Society of Medicine GlaxoSmithKline Fellowship Award for his academic achievements to date and in 2010 Jonathan was awarded a Foreign and Commonwealth Office UK/USA fellowship. In 2012, Jonathan was awarded Royal Society of Medicine-Wesleyan Young Trainee of the Year across all medical and surgical specialties. He attained his PhD degree from University College London in 2013.

Jonathan is committed to a career in Academic ENT, with a strong emphasis on teaching, education, research and career development.

Laura M. Cullen MB BS, BSc (Hons), nMRCGP, DFSRH.

Laura is the twin sister of Jonathan Fishman. She qualified from Imperial College, London with a first class honours BSc in Endocrinology.

She undertook her medical rotations at St Mary's Hospital and The Hammersmith Hospital in London, before joining Barnet VTS, where she completed the nMRCGP.

She is now a GP Partner in North London, with a special interest in teaching and education.

This book is dedicated to our mother, father,
sister and spouses for all their support.

Introduction
and how to use this book

It is a well known fact amongst medical students and doctors alike that 90% of all diagnoses come from the history alone. This concept has been long recognised by generations of practising clinicians, and it is because of this that history-taking is one of the first key principles taught at medical school. For the diagnostician the history carries even more weight nowadays in light of the huge recent advances in laboratory and radiological tests. An (almost) infinite number of tests have become available to the practising clinician, and without a good history and a clear working diagnosis it has become difficult to select the relevant and appropriate tests. It is clearly neither feasible, nor appropriate, to subject any individual patient to a battery of tests in order to make a diagnosis. This is because it is unreliable (false-positive and negative results), time consuming, expensive and potentially harmful (eg in the case of radiation exposure). The history is therefore centre stage in making a correct diagnosis, so that patients can be reliably educated about their condition and managed successfully.

In view of the importance of history taking in the medical school curriculum and in continued medical education, we previously chose to dedicate an entire book to the subject of history taking. Although most current textbooks discuss history taking in a general context, as in our chapter 'The structural basis of history taking', we have decided to shape the acquisition of history-taking skills around certain core topics, which are not only common presentations amongst patients in both general practice and hospital settings, but are also topics frequently encountered by students and doctors in undergraduate and postgraduate examinations. In addition, because patients present to their doctors with symptoms, rather than with diseases, this book adopts a unique symptoms-based approach rather than the classic disease-based approach. This is an entirely new approach in medical education.

For each presenting symptom we have given the types of question that the doctor or student should ask when taking the history from a patient. That is not to say that all histories should conform to a definite, consistent structure every time, but rather to highlight the sort of information that should be gathered from the patient, either through open-ended discussion, or through direct questioning, to reach a correct diagnosis. Indeed, history taking should still be seen as a fluid, patient-led, doctor-steered exercise that cannot be learnt in a robotic fashion. However, this book would be particularly useful in examination preparation, in addition to being a useful adjunct on the wards, as in the former high-pressured scenario the student or doctor is usually expected to make a rapid diagnosis, in just a few minutes, based on the history alone.

At the end of each chapter we have included sections on differential diagnosis and investigations for the particular presenting complaint. We have chosen to highlight in bold those diagnoses that are important not to miss, either because of their clinical significance or because forgetting them may lead to failure of an examination. The investigations section is by no means an exhaustive list and rests on the findings of the history. The investigations selected by the reader should be an accurate reflection of the history and should be chosen to determine which of the differential diagnoses is most accurate.

This book is designed to be used as an adjunct on the wards prior to and while seeing patients, as well as after seeing patients, to provide a prompt, as well ensuring that key questions are not missed. To help in this way, we have dedicated the last section of the book to 'Case scenarios'. Pairs of students or doctors can use these to practise history-taking skills when preparing for examinations or as an aid to training. We have designed them to be challenging but as realistic as possible. The initial introduction, which may be a GP referral letter, is followed by enough information for two students or doctors to role-play an entire history so that the diagnostician can attempt to reach a particular diagnosis.

We are delighted that this book is now in its third edition and we would like to thank all our readers for their comments and suggestions regarding the previous edition. This third edition includes additional chapters and case scenarios, as well as updates throughout the text.

In direct response to feedback, we have also chosen to include a section on 'Asking difficult questions', because some particular questions that deal with sensitive but important issues (such as taking a sexual history) need to be approached in as thoughtful a manner as possible if the diagnostician is to extract the information relevant to the patient's presenting complaint. Most students and doctors admit to finding this a particularly difficult aspect of history taking.

We hope you like the rationale behind this book and what we have tried to achieve. Indeed, much of the book has been designed and developed around and in direct response to student and doctor feedback. We are optimistic that we have created an innovative text that will make a real contribution to current and future medical education.

Jonathan Fishman and Laura Cullen

Abbreviations

AAA	abdominal aortic aneurysm
AAFB	acid–alkali-fast bacillus (TB)
ACE(I)	angiotensin-converting enzyme (inhibitor)
AF	atrial fibrillation
AIDS	acquired immune deficiency syndrome
ALP	alkaline phosphatase
ALT	alanine transaminase
ANA	antinuclear antibodies
ANCA	antineutrophil cytoplasmic antibodies
AP	antero-posterior
APTT	activated partial thromboplastin time
ARF	acute renal failure
AS	ankylosing spondylitis
AST	aspartate transaminase
ATN	acute tubular necrosis
AV	atrioventricular
AVM	arteriovenous malformation
AXR	abdominal X-ray
BAL	bronchoalveolar lavage
BET	benign essential tremor
BM	blood Multistix (instant glucose)
BP	blood pressure
BPH	benign prostatic hypertrophy
BPPV	benign paroxysmal positional vertigo
Ca^{2+}	calcium
CAPD	continuous ambulatory peritoneal dialysis
CCF	congestive cardiac failure
CEA	carcino-embryonic antigen
CMV	cytomegalovirus
CNS	central nervous system
COPD	chronic obstructive pulmonary disease
CPK	creatine (phospho)kinase
CREST	calcinosis raynaud's phenomenon, (o)esophageal dysmotility, sclerodactyly and telangiectasia
CRF	chronic renal failure
CRP	C-reactive protein
CSF	cerebrospinal fluid
CT	computed tomography
CTPA	CT pulmonary angiogram
CTU	CT urogram
CVA	cerebrovascular accident
CXR	chest X-ray
D+V	diarrhoea and vomiting
DEXA	dual-energy X-ray absorptiometry
DIC	disseminated intravascular coagulation
DKA	diabetic ketoacidosis
DM	diabetes mellitus
DMSA	dimercaptosuccinic acid
ds-DNA	double-stranded DNA
DU	duodenal ulcer
DVT	deep vein thrombosis
EAA	extrinsic allergic alveolitis
EBV	Epstein–Barr virus
ECG	electrocardiogram
EEG	electroencephalography
EMG	electromyography
ENA	extractable nuclear antigen
ERCP	endoscopic retrograde cholangio-pancreatography
ESR	erythrocyte sedimentation rate
ETT	exercise tolerance test
FB	foreign body
FBC	full blood count
FHx	family history
FNAC	fine-needle aspiration cytology

FSH	follicle-stimulating hormone	ITP	idiopathic/immune thrombocytopenic purpura
G+S	group and save		
GA	general anaesthetic	IUCD	intrauterine contraceptive device
GCA	giant cell arteritis		
GGT	γ-glutamyl transpeptidase	IVC	inferior vena cava
		IVDU	intravenous drug user
GI	gastrointestinal	IVU	intravenous urography
GN	glomerulonephritis	LDH	lactate dehydrogenase
GORD	gastro-oesophageal reflux disease	LFT	liver function test
		LH	luteinising hormone
GP	general practitioner	LMN	lower motor neurone
GTN	glyceryl trinitrate	LMP	last menstrual period
Hb	haemoglobin	LN	lymphadenopathy/lymph nodes
HbA1c	glycosylated haemoglobin		
		LOC	loss of consciousness
β-hCG	human chorionic gonadotrophin	LP	lumbar puncture
		LRTI	lower respiratory tract infection
HGV	heavy/large goods vehicle		
		LV	left ventricular
HHT	hereditary haemorrhagic telangiectasia	LVF	left ventricular failure
		LVH	left ventricular hypertrophy
5-HIAA	5-hydroxyindoleacetic acid		
		MAO(I)	monoamine oxidase (inhibitor)
HIV	human immunodeficiency virus		
		M,C+S	microscopy, culture and sensitivity
HOCM	hypertrophic obstructive cardiomyopathy		
		MCV	mean cell volume
HPC	history of presenting complaint	MI	myocardial infarction
		MRCP	magnetic resonance cholangio-pancreatography
HPV	human papilloma virus		
HRT	hormone replacement therapy	MRI	magnetic resonance imaging
HSP	Henoch–Schönlein purpura	MS	multiple sclerosis
		MSU	mid-stream specimen of urine
HSV	herpes simplex virus		
HUS	haemolytic-uraemic syndrome	MUGA	multiple-gated acquisition
IBD	inflammatory bowel disease	N+V	nausea and vomiting
		nAChR	nicotinic acetylcholine receptor
IBS	irritable bowel syndrome		
		NPC	nasopharyngeal carcinoma
ICP	intracranial pressure		
IE	infective endocarditis	NPH	normal-pressure hydrocephalus
IGF	insulin-like growth factor		
		NSAID	non-steroidal anti-inflammatory drug
IHD	ischaemic heart disease		
IMB	intermenstrual bleeding	OA	osteoarthritis
INR	international normalised ratio	OCP	oral contraceptive pill

ODQ	on direct questioning		SAH	subarachnoid haemorrhage
OGD	oesophago-gastroduodenoscopy		SCC	squamous cell carcinoma
OM	otitis media		SE	systemic enquiry
OSA	obstructive sleep apnoea		SHx	social history
OTC	over-the-counter		SIADH	syndrome of inappropriate antidiuretic hormone (secretion)
PAN	polyarteritis nodosa		SLE	systemic lupus erythematosus
Pap	Papanicolaou (smear)			
PBC	primary biliary cirrhosis		SOB	short(ness) of breath
PC	presenting complaint		SOL	space occupying lesion
PCB	post-coital bleeding		SPECT	single-photon emission computed tomography
PCOS	polycystic ovarian syndrome		SSRI	serotonin selective reuptake inhibitor
PD	Parkinson's disease			
PE	pulmonary embolism		STI	sexually transmitted infection
PET	positron emission tomography		TB	tuberculosis
PID	pelvic inflammatory disease		TCA	tricyclic antidepressant
			TED	thromboembolic deterrent (stockings)
PMB	post-menopausal bleeding		TFT	thyroid function test
PMHx	past medical history		TIA	transient ischaemic attack
PMR	polymyalgia rheumatica			
PND	paroxysmal nocturnal dyspnoea		TIBC	total iron-binding capacity
PO	per oral		TMJ	temporomandibular joint
PPI	proton pump inhibitor			
PR	per rectum		TSH	thyroid-stimulating hormone
PRN	pro re nata (when required)			
PSA	prostate-specific antigen		TT	thrombin time
PSC	primary sclerosing cholangitis		TTP	thrombotic thrombocytopenic purpura
PSV	public service vehicle/passenger-carrying vehicle		TURP	transurethral resection of the prostate
			UC	ulcerative colitis
PT	prothrombin time		U+Es	urea and electrolytes
PTC	percutaneous transhepatic cholangiography		UMN	upper motor neurone
			USS	ultrasound scan
			UTI	urinary tract infection
PUD	peptic ulcer disease		V/Q	ventilation/perfusion
PV	per vaginam		VDRL	Venereal Disease Research Laboratory (test for syphilis)
RCC	renal cell carcinoma			
RA	rheumatoid arthritis			
RIND	reversible ischaemic neurological deficit		vs	versus
			vWD	von Willebrand's disease
RTA	road traffic accident		WCC	white cell count
RUQ	right upper quadrant			

Italics have been used to highlight questions that you should have in the back of your mind when taking a history.

We have highlighted in **bold** those diagnoses that are important **not** to miss, either because of their clinical significance or because forgetting them could lead to failure of an examination.

The structural basis of history taking

History taking remains and will always remain one of the most fundamental aspects of clinical medicine. The reasons for this are fivefold.

First and foremost, without a good history it is an inevitable fact that the patient's problem will remain undiagnosed, despite examination findings and the results of investigations that follow. Worse still, due to the inherent inaccuracies present in all investigations, of any kind, the clinician who relies solely on the results of investigations may lead to a patient being labelled with an incorrect diagnosis, the implications of which may be profound. The history is therefore pivotal in making a **correct diagnosis**, and the *raison d'être* behind making a correct diagnosis cannot be emphasised enough. Without a diagnosis the cause (**aetiology**), **treatment options** and expected outcome (**prognosis**) of the patient's symptoms will almost certainly remain a complete mystery to the patient and all parties involved in the care of the patient.

Second, the weight attributed to various examination findings and the investigations ultimately selected, along with the way they are interpreted (**post-test probability**), will depend on a good history with a clear working diagnosis (**pre-test probability**). The purpose of the examination and investigations is simply to confirm or refute a specified diagnosis, or hypothesis, made on the basis of the history. Third, the history gives the doctor the unique opportunity to ask about other factors, possibly unrelated to the patient's presenting symptoms, that may have an impact on their future health and of educating them accordingly – so called **opportunistic health promotion**. A good example is smoking. Fourth, a complete history will enable the clinician to assess the impact of the clinical condition on the patient's daily life and will therefore enable them to give medical advice within the context of the patient's social circumstances. Finally, one must never forget the **therapeutic** effect that the doctor–patient interview may have on the patient's psychological state and on the way they view their illness.

The art of taking a good history clearly differs from everyday conversation in that:

- The history requires a clear **rehearsed** structure and a **systematic** approach. It is essential that each of the separate parts comprising the full history is covered carefully in turn. It is the failure to do so, and the omission of whole sections such as the family or drug history, or forgetting to ask particular questions such as drug allergies, that leads to failure in an examination.

- Particular attention should be paid by the doctor to their use of **non-verbal** cues in addition to verbal ones (ie observation, reception, listening, eye contact, silence, gestures, facial expression, posture and position, room layout, etc).
- The doctor is expected to steer the interview conversation to more relevant aspects concerning the patient's presenting complaint, initiating the interview with open questions but then focusing the history and progressing to more closed/direct questions to test a specific diagnosis or hypothesis (**hypothetico-deductive reasoning**).
- The doctor may have to change their use of language, depending on the patient's age and cognitive capacity.

It is the first of the points listed above (the structural basis of history taking) that we shall focus on in this chapter.

The hardest part of taking a history is knowing how to begin. You may find it useful, as we did, to prepare an opening paragraph so that you feel comfortable and give the impression of confidence.

Below is an example of how a history could begin:

Hi/Good morning. I am .... (name), a medical student/doctor, and I'd like to ask you some questions about your illness/condition if I may. (Are you comfortable there before we begin?)

Can you tell me what your name is? It's Mr/Mrs .... isn't it?

How old are you please/and you are .... years old? Is that correct?

What do you do/did you do for a living?

Would you mind telling me, please, what has been the main trouble recently?

OR

So why have you come to see me today, please?

OR

Perhaps you could start, please, by telling me the main problem that has led you to come to hospital?

OR

Could you (start by) tell(ing) me what the problem is please?

Or, if a referral:

> I am .... (name), a medical student/doctor. Your GP, (Dr ....)
> has written to me explaining that you have some trouble with your
> .... I would like to ask you some questions, if I may, so that we
> can decide on a plan of action to investigate this problem? Is that
> OK? Are you comfortable there before we begin?
>
> First of all, can you tell me what your name is/can I just confirm that
> you are Mr/Mrs .... ?
>
> How old are you please? What do you do for a living?
>
> Could you please tell me about the (problem) and how it all started?
>
> This may be followed by: When were you last completely well?

What follows is a generalised template for history taking, which can be
used for any scenario which a medical student/doctor may encounter
during his or her training. It should be memorised early on so that
your history taking is organised. All the focused histories mentioned
throughout this book are based on a similar format. Do try to avoid
medical jargon when interacting with patients. For example, many
patients do not understand the meaning of the term 'reflux', even though
it is very familiar to all those who work within the medical profession (a
better term to use in such an instance would be 'heartburn'). The drug,
social and family histories below are much more detailed and can be
applied to all scenarios later in the book.

The systemic enquiry should be added at the end of all your history
taking and so it is only mentioned here.

➤ Presenting complaint (PC)

What is the problem?

What made you go to the doctor?

Let the patient explain in their own words/expressions and let them
do most of the talking before interrupting. Record the information as
objectively as possible **without interpretation** and, if necessary, quote
the patient directly. Thus a patient presents with 'vomiting up blood', not
haematemesis.

➤ History of presenting complaint (HPC)

When did the problem start?

What made you notice the problem?

How has it progressed since?

Previous history of the problem.

Now **SOCRATES**...

> **S** Site
>
> **O** Onset (sudden/gradual)
>
> **C** Character (dull/sharp/stabbing etc)
>
> **R** Radiation*
>
> **A** Associated symptoms ('What else did you notice?')
>
> **T** Time course/duration
>
> **E** Exacerbating and relieving factors
>
> **S** Severity (on a scale of 1 to 10, with 10 being the worst pain ever experienced, eg childbirth, severe enough to take your own life)
>
> * This is specific to pain, unlike all other components of SOCRATES, which can be applied to any history.

Take a full history of any investigations performed/treatment received for the current condition and response, if any.

Ask about risk factors, if relevant, relating to the presenting problem.

What do you think is wrong with you? It is important to ask the patient this question directly!

What are your **concerns**, **ideas** and **expectations** about the problem?

Patient's **concerns**: What is it about the problem that worries you most?

Patient's **ideas**: What do you think is the cause of your problem?

Patient's **expectations**: What do you think I should do about your problem today?

Effects of the problem: How is this problem affecting your life at the moment?

➤ Past medical history (PMHx)

Current (**active**) and **inactive** medical conditions.

Screen for **MITJTHREADS**: I just need to ask you some routine questions that I ask every patient. Please do not be alarmed in any way by these.

Have you ever had:

Myocardial **I**nfarction, **T**hromboembolism*, **J**aundice, **T**uberculosis, **H**ypertension, **R**heumatic fever, **E**pilepsy, **A**sthma, **D**iabetes, **S**troke?

* Do not forget to screen for clots in the leg and clots in the lung.

Is there any history of previous hospital admissions/operations/illnesses?

If so, when (year), why, how was the diagnosis made, where (which hospital?) and who were you under?

➤ Drug history (DHx)

What medications are you currently taking?

What dose?

Are you taking any tablets or have you had any injections?

Why are you on that?

Compliance – Do you take your medication(s)? (Ask the patient or a carer/relative of the patient). A good way to ask about this is as follows: 'I realise a lot of people don't take all their tablets. Do you have any problems taking yours?'

Side-effects experienced from medication.

Over-the-counter (OTC)/herbal remedies.

Allergies (If so, what happens?).

Vaccinations (Have you had them? Are they up to date?).

➤ Family history (FHx)

Draw a family tree (if relevant).

What relatives do you have?

Are your parents still alive and well? If not, how old were they when they died? What did they die from? Did they suffer from any significant illnesses? Remember siblings, as well as parents, grandparents and children!

Have you any siblings, children, grandchildren?

Are there any diseases or illnesses that 'run in the family'?

Is there history of any consanguinity? Ask about sickle cell disease in all black patients and thalassaemia in all Mediterranean patients.

NB: A **positive** family history may result from shared **genes** or from a shared **environment**.

➤ Social history (SHx)

Smoking

Do you smoke? What do you smoke? Cigarettes/pipe/cigars?

How many do you smoke a day? For how long have you been smoking?

> Cigarette smoking can be quantified as pack-years, where:
>
> Number of pack-years = (packs smoked/day) x (number of years smoked)
>
> One pack contains 20 cigarettes. Thus, 1 pack-year, for example, is equal to smoking 20 cigarettes (1 pack) a day for one year.

Have you tried to stop? Alone or with the help of nicotine replacement therapy/bupropion? How did you get on? What measures helped or hindered your success?

Are you exposed to passive smoking at home?

If the patient does not currently smoke – Have you ever smoked? When did you stop? Why did you stop? ('Why did you stop?' is a particularly useful question in exam situations and may give the answer to the case, eg 'Because of my lung cancer, doc!')

Congratulate the patient for stopping successfully. Empathise with them that from what you hear you understand this is a very difficult thing to do and reinforce the importance of permanent cessation. Brief advice (up to 5 minutes) encouraging patients to make an attempt to quit is effective in promoting smoking cessation (3% quit rate compared with 1% for controls). The essential features of brief opportunistic advice may be remembered with the help of the **5 As**:

Ask about current smoking status (and record). This includes asking about whether other household members smoke.

Advise smokers to stop and explain the health (and physical, social and cosmetic) benefits of doing so.

Assess willingness and motivation to quit.

Assist the smoker to stop (set a date to stop, identification of and strategies to avoid trigger situations; encouragement to develop support from family and friends; ask whether other household members or friends will also consider stopping; suggest finding a partner to quit with for mutual support; consideration of either nicotine replacement or bupropion).

Arrange follow-up or review and refer to local smoking cessation services.

Alcohol

How much alcohol do you consume and how often?

Remember the **CAGE** questionnaire:

Do you ever feel you ought to **c**ut down on your drinking?

Do you get **a**nnoyed when other people tell you to stop drinking?

Do you ever felt **g**uilty about your drinking behaviour?

Have you ever had a drink first thing in the morning to overcome a hangover? (An **e**ye opener)

Two or more positive replies identifies problem drinkers; **one** is an indication for further enquiry about the person's drinking.

Drug abuse

Do you use or have you ever used recreational drugs?

What are the health, social and financial implications of drug misuse?

How do you take them? How frequently and for how long?

Sexual history (if relevant)

I need to ask you some important but rather personal questions, if I may, which may or may not relate to the symptoms you've been having. Is that OK with you?

Are you currently sexually active?

Do you have a regular partner? (Number of partners and for how long?) Have you slept with someone different recently?

Have you engaged in any risky practices? Have you had unprotected sex recently?

For men: Have you ever had sex with another man?

For women: Have you ever had sex with a man known to be bisexual?

Occupation

What is your job now? What does that actually involve doing?

What other jobs have you done? What job have you done the longest?

Have you taken time off work? How much?

Has there been any occupational exposure, such as exposure to dusts, fumes or asbestos?

What are the lifestyle and occupational limitations due to disease?

What is the effect of work on your symptoms? What is the effect of symptoms on your work?

Do you enjoy your current job?

Exercise capacity

Number of stairs able to climb/number of footsteps?

What have your illnesses prevented you from doing?

Overseas travel history

Ask about tropical illnesses.

Have you been abroad in the last year? Where to?

Was prophylaxis (eg against malaria) continued on return?

Animals

Do you keep any pets at home? What are they? Are they well?

Have you had any contact with other animals?

Hobbies

How do you normally spend your days, eg reading, watching TV?

Do you ever go to a day centre?

Home circumstances

Who do you live with?

Do you have any children?

Are you married or single? Is your partner well? What is their job?

Who is at home with you and are they able to look after you?

Who are the most important people in your life?

Who else is at home?

How has your illness affected your spouse, family?

Do you have access to hot water, heating, electricity, or a telephone at home?

Home assistance

Are you normally functionally independent?

What help do you receive? Who are your main carers – relatives, neighbours, friends, social services, support workers, occupational therapists, district nurse?

What modifications, if any, have been made to your house?

What sort of house do you live in (house, flat, bungalow, nursing home)? What floor is your flat on? Is it warden-controlled?

How many levels does your house have? Do you have stairs at home? Do you use the front or back door? Do you have stairs leading to the door?

Is your bedroom upstairs/downstairs? Do you have to climb stairs to reach the toilet? Do you have any rails? Where? In the bedroom/bathroom/on stairs?

Try to ascertain what the patient can do for themselves:

- Can you bathe/shower yourself without assistance? Can you get in and out of the bath easily? Can you use the toilet without assistance?
- How long does it take to dress yourself? Do you need help with dressing? Can you tie your shoes/make a tie/do up buttons/put on a bra, for example, by yourself?
- Who does your shopping? Can you feed yourself and cook for yourself? What do you eat normally? Do you have meals-on-wheels? Can you open tins, bottles or cartons yourself? Do you have trouble peeling potatoes?
- Who does your washing?
- Who does the housework?

Finances

Ask about financial difficulties, social support, state benefits, pension – who collects it?

Other relevant benefits (unemployment/incapacity/disability etc).

Mobility

Try to assess the disabilities:

Do you get out of the house much?

Do you drive?

What was/is your mobility normally like before/now?

How many falls have you had in the last year?

Do you walk unaided or with a walking aid? What do you use? (Stick, Zimmer frame, etc) Do you need a wheelchair to get around?

How far can you usually walk? (On the flat, incline, or in terms of the number of flights of stairs the patient is able to climb) What stops you?

What effect does the illness have on your life? What would you like to do that you can't do or what has your condition prevented you from doing?

How do the symptoms interfere with your life?

Contact with illnesses

Have you been in contact with any person who had tuberculosis or any other infection (eg meningitis, gastroenteritis)?

➤ Systemic enquiry (SE)

Ask about the following symptoms and features:

General – well/unwell, weight (How much have you lost and over how long?), appetite, fevers, (night) sweats, fatigue, recent trauma, lumps, sleep.

Cardiology – chest pain, shortness of breath (When?), orthopnoea/ paroxysmal nocturnal dyspnoea (Do you ever wake up short of breath? How many pillows do you sleep with?), ankle swelling, palpitations (tap out), collapse/dizzy spells/postural hypotension, exercise tolerance, claudication (Do you get pain in your calves when you walk?).

Respiratory – sinusitis, hoarseness, breathlessness, cough (Is it productive?), wheeze, sputum, haemoptysis (How much?), exercise tolerance (metres/number of stairs).

Gastroenterology – mouth ulcers, indigestion, dysphagia, jaundice, nausea, vomiting, haematemesis, diarrhoea (how often, describe), constipation, abdominal pain, masses, rectal bleeding (mixed in or on paper?), change in bowel habit.

Neurology – FFF (fits, faints, funny turns), pins and needles, numbness, difficulty walking, headaches, weakness, unsteadiness, vertigo, co-ordination, tremor, vision, smell, hearing, taste, sphincter disturbances (bladder, bowel, sexual dysfunction), speech, memory, higher mental functions (How do you feel in your spirits?). 'Do your arms and legs work well?' is a good screening aid in neurological assessment.

Genitourinary – dysuria, frequency, nocturia, haematuria, incontinence, hesitancy, poor stream, offensive smell, terminal dribbling, menstrual cycle, sexual function.

Rheumatology – weakness, stiffness, joint pain/swelling, mobility, diurnal variation, functional deficit (Can you dress without help? Can you walk up and down stairs without help?).

Skin – rash, lumps, itch, bruising, hair changes, moles.

Endocrinology – Do you prefer hot/cold weather? Other symptoms covered above.

Gynaecology – periods (heavy, painful). Is there a possibility that you could be pregnant? First day of LMP, IMB/PCB/PMB, vaginal bleeding/discharge, endometriosis, previous recurrent abortions, age of menarche/menopause, previous pregnancies and problems encountered.

Finish with:

Is there anything else that you would like to tell me that I haven't asked you about already?

Do you have any questions before we finish?

Is there anything that you are worried about?

Finally summarise the key points of the history back to the patient. This can be helpful for several reasons:

- Ensures accuracy of your history taking.
- Reassures the patient that you have listened and assimilated the story correctly.
- Helps to cement the story in your own mind.

How to present the history

Practice and good structural technique is the key to making the presentation of the history smooth and concise. It is essential that the key elements of the history are presented and irrelevance is omitted. Again, this comes with practice. Being succinct is crucial, such as when you are on the phone with your seniors in the middle of the night – they will only want the key facts. Below is a template which you may find helpful to form the structural basis of your history presentation:

> .... (name), a .... year-old (age) .... (occupation), with known .... (significant past medical history should be mentioned in the first sentence) was admitted via .... (mode of presentation) .... days ago complaining of a .... (presenting complaint in patient's own words, which is a symptom and not a sign or diagnosis) of .... in duration (time factor).
>
> The history of the present illness began .... ago when he noticed .... (at this point one needs to start from the beginning of the history related to this current episode and it should be chronological, working towards the present admission. One should include SOCRATES and all medical input related to this symptom, including hospital stays, investigations undertaken and medications).
>
> After going through the history of the presenting complaint it is vital at this point to give a list of all the POSITIVE and NEGATIVE risk factors relating to this current episode. For chest pain, for example, this would include hypertension, hypercholesterolaemia, diabetes mellitus, smoking, family history, previous heart disease, stroke or peripheral vascular disease.
>
> The majority of the time should be spent on the above. One can then briefly mention past medical history, drug history with allergies, family history, social history and any relevant findings on direct questioning.

At this point one needs to discuss the positive and relevant negative findings on examination. Conventionally, one starts with general findings on examination – JACCOL (**j**aundice, **a**naemia, **c**yanosis, **c**lubbing, **o**edema, **l**ymphadenopathy) – and vital signs, followed by findings from the examination of the cardiovascular, respiratory and gastrointestinal systems. Then the neurological examination findings should be presented. Finally, it is important to give a ONE-LINE SUMMARY of the case, eg:

> In summary, he is a 50-year-old smoker who presents with sudden-onset chest pain on a background history of ischaemic heart disease.

A **differential diagnosis** (impression) is then required (with the most likely diagnosis at the top of your list), which leads you nicely to the investigations and management plan.

Example

Joe Bloggs, a 45-year-old retired builder, with known coronary artery disease, was admitted via Accident and Emergency last night with sudden onset of chest pain of 6 hours' duration.

The history of the present illness began 5 years ago when he started getting chest pains on exertion while gardening. He went to see his GP, who referred him to a cardiologist. He was investigated for ischaemic heart disease at this time at St Hugh's Hospital where coronary angiography and angioplasty were undertaken. Mr Bloggs had been symptom-free up until yesterday when, 5 minutes after returning home from a 5-km run, he experienced sudden-onset, central crushing chest pain which lasted 30 minutes. It radiated down his left arm and up his neck. He had associated difficulty breathing and sweating but he did not lose consciousness. The pain was severe and he graded the pain as 9 out of 10. It was not relieved by his GTN spray. His wife called the ambulance and he was blue-lighted into hospital.

Mr Bloggs has smoked 20 cigarettes a day for 25 years, and takes a statin for his hypercholesterolaemia, which was diagnosed 5 years ago. He is not diabetic, not hypertensive and has never had a stroke, TIA or peripheral vascular disease. There is a strong family history, with Mr Blogg's brother dying of an MI at the age of 47 and his father dying of a stroke at 65.

In Mr Bloggs' past medical history, he had an appendicectomy when he was 16 years old. He has never had jaundice, TB, PE or DVT, hypertension, rheumatic fever, epilepsy or asthma (MITJTHREADS).

Mr Bloggs is currently on atorvastatin 40 mg once a day, aspirin 75 mg once a day. He has never been thrombolysed and has no known drug allergies.

In his social history, Mr Bloggs used to run his own building company until 5 years ago when he was diagnosed as having ischaemic heart disease. He is now retired. He lives with his wife and two children in a house and is usually very active, managing to run 5–10 km once a week without any difficulties. He drinks 4 units of alcohol a week and does not take recreational drugs. On direct questioning, Mr Bloggs explained that he has lost 7 kg of weight in the last 3 months.

On examination last night, Mr Bloggs appeared uncomfortable, sweaty and breathless. There was no evidence of jaundice, anaemia, cyanosis, clubbing, oedema or lymphadenopathy. His BP was 100/55, pulse 100/min and his temperature was 38 degrees. On examination of his cardiovascular system, the jugular venous pressure (JVP) was raised by 4 cm, and heart sounds 1 and 2 were present. There was a 5/6 pansystolic murmur, loudest over the apex, radiating to the axilla. There were no additional heart sounds. There were no carotid bruits and there was evidence of pitting ankle oedema up to the knees.

On examination of the respiratory system, respiration rate was 20 beats/min with saturations of 98% on 4 litres of oxygen via a bag and mask. There was good bilateral lung expansion and the lungs were dull to percussion at the bases. There was good bilateral air entry on auscultation with bibasal fine inspiratory crackles. The abdomen was soft and not tender with no evidence of scars or organomegaly. Bowel sounds were present and normal. Cranial nerves were grossly intact and the peripheral nervous system was normal.

In summary, Mr Bloggs is a 45-year-old smoker with known ischaemic heart disease who now presents with an acute episode of chest pain and breathlessness, with evidence of heart failure and mitral regurgitation on examination. My differential diagnosis is as follows:

Myocardial infarction

Pulmonary embolus

Pneumothorax

Aortic dissection

Abdominal masses and distension

➤ History of presenting complaint

When did the lump appear?

SOCRATES

Site

Where is the lump?

Onset

Duration?

How was it noticed and by whom? (suddenly appeared, painful).

Have your clothes become tighter recently?

Character

Is it focal or generalised?

Associated symptoms

Is it producing local symptoms?

Is there pain or discomfort?

Are there any other lumps?

Are there any systemic symptoms (weight loss, malaise, change in bowel habit, anorexia, fever?).

➤ The 7 F's

*Are there any symptoms of bowel obstruction (**F**latus)?* – colicky abdominal pain, vomiting, absolute constipation, abdominal distension. Are there any changes in bowel habit or rectal bleeding? (think about the causes of bowel obstruction).

*Is there any shortness of breath due to **F**luid accumulation, or ascites, (causing splintage of the diaphragm)? Are there any features suggesting liver disease and in particular portal hypertension eg jaundice, haematemesis (varices), dilated veins on abdomen, rectal bleeding (haemorrhoids). Are there any signs of jaundice or symptoms of anaemia?*

Are you constipated? (**F**aeces)

Have you put on weight recently? (**F**at)

Is there any chance that you could be pregnant? (**F**etus)

Are there any symptoms of malabsorption eg steatorrhoea (Are your stools pale, bulky, offensive? Do your stools float? Are they difficult to flush away?) (**F**ood – coeliac disease causes abdominal distension).

Are there any Gynaecological/Genitourinary symptoms? – dysuria, frequency, urgency, urge incontinence, haematuria, vaginal bleeding (**F**lipping Great Masses). Is there any associated leg swelling/ DVTs/ varicosities (extrinsic venous compression)?

Timing/duration

Is it enlarging/staying the same/getting smaller? Over what time course?

What do you think is wrong?

Is there anything that you are worried this might be due to?

Ask about treatment, if any, already received?

➤ Past medical history

MITJTHREADS

Is there any history of previous hospital admissions/operations/illnesses, especially abdominal disorders or operations?

Is so when (year), why, how was the diagnosis made, where (which hospital?), who were you under?

Is there a history of IBD?

Is there a history of any gynaecological problems (flipping great masses) such as fibroids, ovarian cysts etc.

Is there any history of known hernias, maldescended testes, or AAA?

➤ Drug history

What medications are you currently taking?

What dose?

Why are you on that?

Compliance, side-effect(s) of medication, OTC/herbal remedies, allergies. (What happens?)

➤ Social history

To focus on:

- Smoking
- Alcohol
- Recreational drugs
- Overseas travel history such as hydatid cysts
- Occupation (heavy lifting → hernias)

Lifestyle limitations due to disease.

Has patient taken time off work? How much?

What are your hobbies?

How do the symptoms interfere with your life (walking, working, sleeping)?

➤ Family history

Are there any diseases or illnesses that 'run in the family'?

Is there a FHx of malignancy, especially bowel carcinoma?

Has there been any contact with TB or other infections?

Is there a FHx of polycystic kidney disease?

Is there any consanguinity? Draw a family tree.

➤ Differential diagnosis

- Fat (Obesity)
- Fetus (Pregnancy)
- Flatus (Air)
  - **Bowel Obstruction**
  - Aerophagy (air swallowing) eg IBS
- Fluid (Ascites)
  - Chronic peritonitis (eg TB, missed appendicitis)
  - Carcinomatosis (malignant deposits especially ovarian, stomach)
  - Chronic liver disease (cirrhosis, secondary deposits, portal or hepatic vein obstruction, parasitic infections)
  - Congestive heart failure (right-sided)
  - Chronic renal failure (nephrotic syndrome)
  - Chyle (lymphatic duct disruption)
  - Constrictive pericarditis
- Faeces
  - Chronic constipation
  - Chronic intestinal obstruction
  - Hirschsprung's disease
  - Acquired megacolon
- Flipping great masses
  - Uterine fibroids
  - Giant Hepatomegaly/splenomegaly
  - Giant renal cell carcinoma
  - Polycystic kidneys
  - Lymph nodes
  - Abdominal aortic aneurysm

- Abdominal cysts – renal, pancreatic, ovarian, pancreatic pseudocyst, mesenteric, hydatid
- Desmoid tumour
- Bladder (retention)
- Food
  - Malabsorption syndromes eg coeliac disease

> Investigations

Blood tests

- Haematology – FBC, ESR, blood film
  - Anaemia (anaemia of chronic disease)
  - Polycythaemia (RCC)
  - Raised WCC (blood dyscrasias, diverticular disease, renal infections, empyema gall bladder etc)
  - ESR (malignancy, chronic inflammation)
  - Blood film (blood dyscrasias and hepatosplenomegaly)
- Biochemistry
  - U+Es (vomiting and dehydration eg gallbladder and bowel lesions, ureteric obstruction, renal lesions)
  - Ca^{2+} (carcinoma)
  - Glucose (pancreatitis, pancreatic carcinoma)
  - CRP (infection)
  - LFTs (liver lesions, metastases, low albumin in ascites)
  - Amylase (pancreatic pseudocyst)
  - PSA (prostate carcinoma)

Urine (M,C&S)

- Haematuria (RCC, bladder tumours)
- Pus cells
- Organisms
- Malignant cells
- β-hCG (pregnancy)

Radiology

- CXR
  - Congestive cardiac failure
  - Metastases
- AXR
  - Bowel obstruction
  - Constipation
  - Large spleen/liver
  - Renal/ureteric calculi
- Transabdominal/transvaginal USS
  - Organomegaly
  - AAA
  - Cysts/collections
  - Enlarged bladder
  - Ovarian/uterine lesions
- CT abdomen ± guided biopsy
  - Carcinoma
  - Collection/cyst

Further investigations

- OGD (carcinoma stomach, pyloric stenosis)
- Small bowel enema (Crohn's, carcinoma)
- Barium enema (carcinoma bowel, diverticular)
- Colonoscopy (carcinoma colon, diverticular)
- Cystoscopy (bladder tumour)
- Paracentesis – If ascites for cytology, culture (microbiology) and protein content (biochemistry)
- Diagnostic laparoscopy ± biopsy

Acute abdominal pain

➤ History of presenting complaint

Site

Can you point with a finger to the location of the pain?

Onset

When did the pain start? Where did it start?

Has it moved since?

What were you doing when the pain started?

How quickly did it come on? (Suddenly, over seconds, minutes, gradually)

Character

Where is the pain worst?

What is the pain like – aching, sharp/stabbing/like a knife, burning?

Is it constant or variable? Is it colicky?

Radiation

Does the pain radiate? (To the back – AAA, pancreatitis; down into the groin/genitals – renal/ureteric colic, testicular torsion; to the shoulders – gallbladder; loin – pyelonephritis; chest – MI)

Associations

What else did you notice?

General

- Sweating/fever
- Rigors
- Shortness of breath
- Dizziness on standing (Concealed/covert haemorrhage)

Gastrointestinal – Have you had any

- Acid reflux, waterbrash?
- Pain during swallowing? (Odynophagia) Difficulty swallowing? (Dysphagia)
- Nausea or vomiting? (Onset, duration, persistence, how much, frequency, composition – blood, bile, small-bowel contents, coffee-grounds)
  - What came first, the vomiting or the pain? (NB: Classically, if pain comes on first, followed by vomiting, this suggests a surgical cause. If vomiting comes on first, followed by pain, this suggests a medical cause for the pain)
  - What effect did vomiting have on the pain?
- *Is there diarrhoea (frequency, consistency, blood/mucus/ pus), constipation, haematemesis/melaena/PR bleeding, painful defecation? Is there any recent change in bowel habit? Are there any symptoms of indigestion, steatorrhoea, or weight loss?*
- *Are there any features of bowel obstruction?*
  - When were your bowels last open?
  - When was flatus last passed?
  - Are you able to pass flatus at the moment?
  - Is there any distension or vomiting?
- *Are there any current hernias?*

Genitourinary – *Are there urinary symptoms?* (Suggestive of UTI or acute retention: ask about frequency, dysuria, urgency, haematuria, nocturia, hesitancy, poor stream, terminal dribbling, etc)

Gynaecology

- Have you had previous gynaecological problems?
- Do you mind me asking if you are sexually active?
- At what stage are you at in your menstrual cycle at the moment? Are there any problems with menstruation?
- *Is there per vaginal bleeding, PID/inflammation of the tubes, ovarian cysts?*
- When was the first day of your last menstrual period? (Menses – duration, regular, heavy, painful; PV discharge; PV bleeding; IMB, PCB, PMB; fibroids; endometriosis; relation of pain to menstrual cycle (mittelschmerz))
- Is it possible you could be pregnant? (Ectopic)
- Has there been recent trauma? (Delayed rupture of spleen!)

Timing

What is the duration? (> 6 hours of unremitting pain is likely to be surgical rather than medical)

Have you had it before? If so, how was it different?

When does the pain occur and how frequently?

Exacerbating/relieving factors

What brings it on/what made the pain worse?

What relieves the pain (What takes the pain away)? (Rest, posture/movement/lying flat, analgesia, antacids, milk, defecation)

What brings on the pain?

- Does breathing affect the pain?
- Does breathing deeply make it worse?
- How about coughing, movement, hot drinks, alcohol? (Gastritis, pancreatitis)
- Food? (Fatty foods – the pain of gallbladder pathology, acute pancreatitis, mesenteric ischaemia, PUD and GORD can all be precipitated by food)
- Exercise/exertion?

Severity

Is it the worst pain you have ever experienced? Score out of 10 compared with childbirth or 10 being severe enough to take your own life.

Have you taken time off work or been away from school because of the pain?

Is your sleep affected?

Risk factors

> ### ➤ Risk factors for AAA

Hypertension
Smoking
Advancing age
Family history of AAA
COPD
Cardiac disease
Previous stroke

> ### ➤ Risk factors for pancreatitis (GET SMASHED)

Gallstones and **E**thanol – two commonest causes of pancreatitis
Trauma
Steroids
Mumps
Autoimmune (PAN)
Scorpion bites
Hypothermia, **H**ypercalcaemia, **H**ypertriglyceridaemia
ERCP, **E**mboli
Drugs – thiazides, azathioprine

What do you think is wrong?

Ask about treatment already received (eg NSAIDs).

Acute abdominal pain

➤ Past medical history

Is there history of previous GI disease? (Indigestion, abdominal pain)

Do you suffer from gallstones?

Have you had an AAA, peptic ulcer, diverticular disease or pancreatitis before?

Have you had abdominal surgery previously (adhesions)?

Have you had previous gynaecological problems?

Have you had a previous appendicectomy?

Consider the patient's fitness for general anaesthesia – Have you had any reactions to general anaesthetics in the past?

➤ Drug history

Are you taking any medications, especially:

- Anti-inflammatories? (Cause PUD)
- Steroids? (Mask abdominal signs)
- The pill or HRT? (Need to be stopped prior to surgery due to increased thromboembolic risk)

Compliance, side-effect(s) of medication, OTC/herbal remedies, allergies.

(What happens?)

➤ Social history

Do you smoke? (Important to stop pre-operatively because of increased risk of thrombosis)

Do you drink alcohol? (Gastritis, acute/chronic pancreatitis)

Do you use recreational drugs?

Sexual history – I need to ask you some important though rather personal questions, if I may, which may or may not relate to the symptoms you've been having. Have you had recent unprotected intercourse with a new partner? (PID/salpingitis)

How would you manage at home after a possible operation? Who is at home to look after you on discharge? (The situation at home is very important if considering surgery.)

➤ Family history

Is there a family history of any GI conditions, eg IBD (UC/Crohn's disease)?

Is there a family history of rare metabolic causes of abdominal pain, eg porphyria, familial Mediterranean fever?

Do any anaesthetic reactions run in the family? (Malignant hyperpyrexia syndrome)

➤ Differential diagnosis

Right hypochondrium	Epigastric	Left hypochondrium
Basal pneumonia **Hepatitis** **Gallbladder pathology** **(biliary colic, acute/** **chronic cholecystitis,** **cholangitis)** Congestive hepatomegaly	**Oesophagitis/gastritis** **Peptic ulcer disease** **Gallbladder pathology** **Acute pancreatitis** **Myocardial infarct** **Perforated oesophagus** **(Boerhaave's)** **Abdominal aortic** **aneurysm**	Basal pneumonia **Ruptured spleen** Splenomegaly Splenic infarction Subphrenic abscess
Right loin/flank	**Central/periumbilical**	**Left loin/flank**
Pyelonephritis **Renal/ureteric colic** Renal infarct	**Abdominal aortic** **aneurysm** **Acute pancreatitis** Gastroenteritis **Bowel obstruction** Early appendicitis **Ischaemic bowel** **(mesenteric** **thrombosis)** **Testicular torsion**	**Pyelonephritis** **Renal/ureteric colic** Renal infarct
Right iliac fossa	**Suprapubic**	**Left iliac fossa**
Appendicitis Meckel's diverticulitis Mesenteric adenitis Perforated caecal carcinoma Crohn's disease Terminal ileitis **Renal/ureteric colic** Ovarian cyst accident (rupture, haemorrhage, torsion) **Ectopic pregnancy** Salpingitis **Testicular torsion**	Cystitis/UTI Urinary retention Uterine fibroid (red degeneration)	**Diverticulitis** Constipation **Renal/ureteric colic** **Sigmoid volvulus** **Colitis (ischaemic,** **infective, ulcerative)** Ovarian cyst accident (rupture, haemorrhage, torsion) **Ectopic pregnancy** Salpingitis **Testicular torsion**

Acute abdominal pain

Medical causes of abdominal pain

Cardiovascular

- **Myocardial infarction**
- **Aortic dissection**
- Bornholm's disease (Coxsackie B)

Respiratory

- **Basal pneumonia**

Metabolic

- **Diabetic ketoacidosis**
- **Addisonian crisis**
- **Sickle cell crisis**
- **Hypercalcaemia**
- Uraemia
- Phaeochromocytoma
- Acute intermittent porphyria
- Lead poisoning

Infections

- **Gastroenteritis**
- Tuberculosis
- Typhoid fever
- Malaria
- Cholera
- *Yersinia enterocolitica*
- **Urinary tract infection**

Neurological

- Herpes zoster/shingles (NB: dermatomal)
- Tabes dorsalis

Inflammatory

- Vasculitis
  - HSP
  - PAN
- Familial Mediterranean fever

Psychogenic

- Narcotic addiction
- Irritable bowel syndrome

➤ Investigations

Blood tests

- Haematology – FBC, ESR, clotting, cross-match/G+S
  - Anaemia (bleeding, anaemia of chronic disease)
  - Raised WCC (infection, inflammation)
  - ESR (infection, inflammation, malignancy)
  - Clotting (pre-op prep)
  - Cross-match/G+S (AAA, ectopic, pre-op prep)
- Biochemistry
  - U+Es (vomiting and diarrhoea, renal lesions)
  - CRP (infection)
  - Glucose (DKA, pancreatitis)
  - LFTs (hepatitis, gallstones)
  - Ca^{2+} (pancreatitis, renal colic, hypercalcaemia as a primary cause)
  - Amylase (pancreatitis, ischaemic bowel)
  - Lipids (pancreatitis)
  - β-hCG (ectopic)
- Microbiology
  - Blood cultures (Gram-negative sepsis)
  - Arterial blood gases (pancreatitis, metabolic acidosis)

Urinalysis (M,C+S)

- Pus cells, nitrites, protein, organisms (pyelonephritis, UTI)
- Blood (renal colic)
- β-hCG (ectopic)
- Glucose, ketones (DKA)

ECG

- Exclude MI
- Pre-op preparation for anaesthetic
- Arrhythmias (eg AF) leading to emboli (acutely ischaemic bowel)

Radiology

- Erect CXR
  - Perforated viscus
  - Basal pneumonia
  - Pneumomediastinum (Boerhaave's syndrome)
- AXR (± lateral decubitus)
  - Bowel obstruction
  - Constipation
  - AAA
  - Renal calculi
  - Thumbprinting of bowel wall (bowel ischaemia)
- Transabdominal/transvaginal USS
  - Exclude gynaecological pathology
  - Collection/cyst
  - Free fluid (peritonitis, ascites)
  - AAA
  - Gallstones
  - Renal stones
- CT abdomen/pelvis
  - Collections
  - Anastomotic leak
  - Diverticulitis
  - Renal colic (CTU)
  - Tumours

Acute abdominal pain

Further investigations

- OGD ± biopsy and *Helicobacter pylori* testing (peptic ulcer, malignancy)
- Large-bowel enema/Gastrografin ('instant') enema (cause for large-bowel obstruction)
- Small-bowel enema/follow-through (Crohn's disease)
- Duplex Doppler/angiography (mesenteric thrombosis)
- Diagnostic laparoscopy
- Vaginal/endocervical swabs (PID)
- Blood film/Hb electrophoresis (sickle cell crisis)
- VDRL (tabes dorsalis)
- Urinary porphobilinogens (acute intermittent porphyria)
- Short synacthen test (Addison's disease)

Alcohol-related problems

➤ History of presenting complaint

How **much** do you drink? How much do you drink on each occasion?

How **often** do you drink?

What do you drink?

How many units do you drink in a week? (1 unit = 1 small (125-ml) glass wine, 1 shot (25 ml) whisky, 0.5 pint beer (standard 3.5%))

How **long** does it take you to finish a bottle of whisky/vodka?

> ### ➤ CAGE questionnaire
>
> Have you ever thought that you ought to **c**ut down on your drinking?
>
> Have people **a**nnoyed you by criticising your drinking?
>
> Have you ever felt **g**uilty about your drinking?
>
> Have you ever had a drink first thing in the morning to overcome a hangover? (An **e**ye opener)

Two or more positive replies identifies problem drinkers; **one** is an indication for further enquiry about the person's drinking.

Do you find that you tend to drink more than your friends around you when you are out socialising? Do they ever comment on how much you drink, or ask you to reduce your intake?

How often during the past year have you been unable to remember what happened the night before because you had been drinking?

History

If intake is low risk, ask about any previous history of heavy drinking or dependence.

Age of onset of regular drinking/alcohol misuse/harmful drinking.

Amount

Are you a binge drinker, or do you drink consistently? (If the former is true, ask for how long, how much consumed, how long in between binges and precipitating factors for binges)

How much money do you spend on alcohol?

Place of drinking

Do you drink alone or with other people?

Other

What is the **purpose** of your drinking?

What is your **attitude** towards alcohol?

Do you take any **drugs** as well?

Conditions associated with drinking

- CNS:Wernicke–Korsakoff syndrome, polyneuropathy
- Gastrointestinal: gastritis, pancreatitis, liver disease, carcinoma of oesophagus
- Endocrine: cushingoid face
- Cardiovascular: hypertension, cardiac arrhythmias, cardiomyopathy
- Metabolism: gout
- Musculoskeletal: myopathies

Dependency

What happens when you go without alcohol for long periods of time? (Manifestations of dependency)

Are you aware of your compulsion to drink?

Tolerance

Is your tolerance increasing? Are you able to drink more now than you used to before getting drunk?

Withdrawal symptoms

Do you get withdrawal symptoms if you go without a drink for a long period of time?

When – first thing in the morning?

Do you get shaking, agitation, nausea, retching, sweating?

Are your symptoms relieved by drinking alcohol?

Do you get hallucinations, or altered perceptions?

Counselling/advice/treatments

Ask about previous advice, counselling and treatments received for alcohol problems.

➤ Past medical history

Have you ever had to detoxify?

Were you admitted to hospital or managed at home?

Establish the history and current situation with regard to the following systems:

Gastrointestinal

- Liver disease
- Jaundice
- Pancreatitis
- Abdominal pain
- Gastritis
- GI haemorrhage
- Carcinoma of mouth, oesophagus, liver

Cardiovascular

- Hypertension
- Cardiomyopathy
- Arrhythmias

Neurological

- Neuropathy
- Psychosis
- Memory difficulties
- Hallucinations
- Cognitive impairment
- Blackouts
- Fits
- Accidents
- Anxiety

Respiratory

- Chest infections

Metabolic

- Gout

Reproductive

- Sexual dysfunction
- Fetal alcohol syndrome (in women of reproductive age)

➤ Drug history

Do you take any medications?

Do you take any drugs that may interact with alcohol, eg warfarin, anticonvulsants, disulfiram, metronidazole?

➤ Social history

Do you smoke? (Reinforces drinking behaviour and vice versa)

Do you use recreational drugs?

Have there been any requests for medical certificates?

Has there been any absenteeism at work?

Do you have any marital or family problems and has there been any domestic violence?

Has alcohol ever led you to neglect yourself, your family or work?

Do you have any financial difficulties?

Have you had any prosecutions for violent behaviour or driving offences? Have you ever been done for drink/drunk driving? Have you or someone else been injured as a result of your drinking?

Have you ever had your driving licence taken away or penalty points awarded relating to alcohol misuse?

Family, housing, social and employment situations and the effect of alcohol misuse on these.

Do you receive any state benefits – unemployment, incapacity, disability?

Have you made any attempts to stop drinking? What? When was the last time? How? Why did you fail?

Do you presently attend or have you ever been to Alcoholics Anonymous? Have you heard of it? Have you thought before about going?

➤ Complications of alcohol misuse

Gastrointestinal

- Oesophagus
  - Gastro-oesophageal reflux
  - Oesophageal carcinoma
  - **Oesophageal varices**
  - Mallory–Weiss syndrome
- Stomach
  - Gastritis
  - **Peptic ulcer disease**
- Small intestine
  - Malabsorption and malnutrition
  - Altered motor activity (diarrhoea)

Alcohol-related problems

- Liver
  - Fatty liver (steatosis)
  - **Alcoholic hepatitis**
  - **Liver cirrhosis and its complications**
    - ➤ **Ascites**
    - ➤ **Spontaneous bacterial peritonitis**
    - ➤ **Portal hypertension**
    - ➤ **Hepatocellular carcinoma**
- Spleen
  - Splenomegaly (portal hypertension)
- Pancreas
  - **Pancreatitis** (acute and chronic)
  - Pancreatic carcinoma

Cardiovascular

- **Coronary heart disease**
- Dilated cardiomyopathy
- Hypertension
- Cardiac arrhythmias

Respiratory

- Aspiration pneumonia

Neurological

- **Seizures/uncontrolled epilepsy**
- **Cerebrovascular accidents**
- Cerebellar degeneration (ataxia)
- **Wernicke–Korsakoff syndrome (thiamine deficiency)**
- Peripheral polyneuropathy (mainly sensory)
- **Hypoglycaemic coma**
- **Hepatic encephalopathy**
- Alcoholic dementia
- Marchiafava–Bignami syndrome (corpus callosum atrophy)
- Central pontine myelinolysis
- Myopathy (acute/chronic)
- Rhabdomyolysis
- Neuropraxia

Haematological

- Haemolysis (Zieve's syndrome)
- Impaired erythropoiesis
- Macrocytosis
- Alcoholism-associated folate deficiency
- Sideroblastic anaemia
- Neutropenia
- **Thrombocytopenia**
- **Clotting factor deficiency (liver failure)**
- Warfarin and other drug interactions (liver failure)

Endocrine/metabolic

- Hypoalbuminaemic state
- **Hypoglycaemia**
- Hypogonadism/infertility
- Hyperoestrogenaemia/gynaecomastia
- Pseudo-Cushing's syndrome
- Ketoacidosis
- Gout
- Osteopenia/osteoporosis/fractures

Dermatological

- Facial flushing
- Palmar erythema
- Spider naevi
- Linear telangiectasia
- Dupuytren's contracture
- Caput medusae (portal hypertension)
- Parotid enlargement

Pregnancy

- Infertility
- Fetal alcohol syndrome
- Intrauterine growth retardation
- Increased risk of abortion/stillbirth

Psychiatric

- Alcohol dependency/addiction/misuse
- Alcohol withdrawal
- Acute confusional state
- **Alcohol intoxication** (falls/blackouts/accidents/injuries, dangerous driving, violence, criminal behaviour)
- Alcoholic hallucinosis
- **Delirium tremens**
- Depression and anxiety
- Suicide
- Alcoholic dementia

Social

- Job loss
- Marital/relationship difficulties
- Criminal activity
- Violence
- Driving offences and RTAs

➤ Investigations

Blood tests

- Haematology – FBC, clotting, haematinics
  - Anaemia (multifactorial)
  - Thrombocytopenia (multifactorial)
  - MCV (macrocytosis)
  - Clotting (liver disease)
  - Haematinics (vitamin B_{12}, red cell folate)
- Biochemistry
  - LFTs including GGT (cirrhosis)
  - U+Es (hepatorenal syndrome)
  - Glucose (liver disease, pancreatic failure)
  - Albumin (liver failure)
  - Lipids (secondary hyperlipidaemia)
  - Blood ethanol levels (intoxication)

Radiology

- CXR
  - Large heart (dilated cardiomyopathy)
  - Aspiration
- USS
  - Fatty liver
  - Hepatitis
  - Cirrhosis
  - Evidence of portal hypertension

Further investigations

- Carbohydrate-deficient transferrin (alcoholism)
- Red cell transketolase (Wernicke's)
- Echocardiography (dilated cardiomyopathy)
- OGD (varices, PUD)
- Liver biopsy (liver disease)
- EEG (hepatic encephalopathy)
- Nerve conduction studies (neuropathy)

Ano-rectal pain

➤ History of presenting complaint

Site

Where do you feel the pain? (in the skin or deep inside?)

Onset

Sudden vs gradual

Is it there the whole time or precipitated by something, eg passing stool?

Duration?

Character

Is the pain spasmodic? (proctalgia)

Is it worse during or after defecation (anal fissure)?

Does it persist after defecation?

Associated symptoms

- Are there any other pains, such as abdominal pain?
- Is there any bleeding from the back passage?
- Are there any changes in bowel habit? Is there tenesmus?
- Is there passage of mucus/pus/blood?
- Are there any lumps, or the sensation of something coming down when you pass stools?
- Are you still able to reduce your piles?
- Is there a history of trauma?
- Are you able to pass urine, or is there any back pain or weakness of your legs? (rarely cauda equina lesions present this way).
- Are there any systemic features – weight loss, fever, malaise, anorexia, rigors?

Precipitating factors

- Straining
- Passing stool

Relieving factors

- GTN cream

What do you think is wrong?

Ask about treatment, if any, already received?

➤ Past medical history

MITJTHREADS

Are there any previous illnesses?

Have you had prolapsing piles in the past?

Is there a history of Crohn's disease or TB (chronic perianal sepsis)

➤ Drug history

Do you take any tablets, creams or injections such as GTN, diltiazem, lignocaine creams, botulinum toxin, or laxatives?

➤ Social history

Have you had any time off work because of the problem? How much?

Are you unable to sit down for long periods?

What effect does the pain have on your sleep?

➤ Family history

Is there a FHx of malignancy?

Has there been any contact with TB or other infections?

➤ Differential diagnosis

Acute
- Trauma
- Thrombosed, strangulated haemorrhoids
- Perianal haematoma/thrombosis
- Fissure-in-ano
- Perianal abscess
- Intersphincteric abscess
- Ischiorectal abscess
- Pilonidal abscess/sinus

Chronic
- Fistula-in-ano
- Rectal prolapse
- Ano-rectal malignancy
- Solitary rectal ulcer
- Chronic perianal sepsis, eg Crohn's, TB
- Proctalgia fugax
- Cauda equina lesions

➤ Investigations

Blood tests
- Haematology – FBC, ESR
  - Anaemia (malignancy)
  - Raised WCC (collection)
  - ESR (Crohn's, TB, malignancy)
- Biochemistry
  - U+Es (renal function)
  - CRP (infection)
  - Glucose (diabetes mellitus)
- Microbiology
  - Blood cultures (sepsis)

Proctoscopy (haemorrhoids, ano-rectal malignancy)

Radiology

- MRI
    - Perianal sepsis (to define fistulae)

Further investigations

- Rigid sigmoidoscopy (ano-rectal malignancy)
- Endoanal ultrasound (fistula-in-ano)

Back pain

NB: *Red flag* (more sinister) symptoms, as laid out by the Royal College of General Practitioners, are indicated in bold. *Yellow flags* (social exacerbations) have been incorporated in the social history.

➤ History of presenting complaint

When did the pain start?

What were you doing when the pain started?

Is it progressive and getting worse, the same, or getting better?

Have you had it before? If so, how was it different? Is the pain constant or intermittent?

SOCRATES

Site

Where is the pain?

Is it well localised or diffuse?

Is there any **thoracic pain?**

Does the pain extend below the knee? What percentage of the total pain is back pain and what percentage is leg pain?

Onset

Did the pain start suddenly or gradually?

Is there a history of **trauma** or injury?

Duration?

Character

What is the pain like – aching, sharp/stabbing/like a knife, burning, shooting/radicular?

Is it **constant/persistent** or variable?

Is there persistent limitation of movement in all directions (AS), or only some?

Is there pain at night? If so, does it drive you out of bed in the middle of the night?

Is there pain at rest? Is there morning stiffness? (AS)

Is there any pins and needles or numbness? Where?

Radiation

Does the pain radiate to the abdomen, along the course of the aorta and its branches? (Neck, ear, back, abdomen – AAA/aortic dissection)

Does the pain radiate into the legs/calves? (Sciatica) What about into the groin? (Renal colic)

Associated symptoms

Are there symptoms of:

- Spinal cord compression?
- Disturbance of **bladder** function (urinary incontinence or retention)?
- **Bowel** function (diarrhoea, faecal incontinence, constipation)?
- **Leg weakness** (and is it bilateral)?
- Erectile failure/impotence, sensory disturbances (sensory level, leg numbness, paraesthesia, **saddle anaesthesia around anus, perineum, genitals**)?

Is there significant muscle weakness (3/5 or less), or foot drop (both suggest disc prolapse)? Have you noticed any muscle wasting or fasciculations?

Gait/balance disturbances? Are any other joints involved? (AS etc)

Is your breathing affected?

Are there any pulsatile swellings in the abdomen? (AAA, ask about AAA risk factors – see Acute abdominal pain)

Could this be cord compression/cauda equina syndrome?

Do you have a normal feeling of a full bladder at the moment?

Do you feel urine passing down the urethra? How do you know you have finished passing urine? (The noise?)

Can you currently differentiate between flatus and faeces?

Precipitating factors

Is the pain site tender when you press on it?

Is the pain exacerbated by movement?

When is the pain worse?

Are there any symptoms of sciatica – Do these symptoms increase with straining or coughing?

Is the pain related to movement?

When is the pain worse/better? (Sitting, standing, lying, walking, bending down (such as putting on socks), at night, coughing)

Relieving factors

What relieves the pain – rest, posture, analgesia? What have you tried already?

Severity

Is this the worst pain you have ever had? Score out of 10 (10 being the pain of childbirth, or so bad that they would consider taking their own life because of it).

Try to engage in the severity of the pain by asking questions such as – Does it keep you awake at night, or does it make you stop activities?

Are there any systemic symptoms – **fever**, **rigors**, **malaise**, **weight loss**, eye pain (iritis), skin rashes/psoriasis, colitis/diarrhoea, urethral discharge?

Distinguish spinal claudication/stenosis from vascular claudication by asking when the pain is worst – walking/resting/sitting to standing, bending over, cycling, walking uphill or downhill etc (see Leg pain).

What do you think is wrong?

What are your concerns, ideas and expectations regarding treatment?

Ask about treatment already received (eg NSAIDs)?

➤ Past medical history

MITJTHREADS

Is there any history of back problems/operations?

Is there a history of gallstones/pancreatitis/AAA?

Is there any significant gynaecological history? (Referred pain)

Is there a history of known malignant disease or serious illnesses such as arthritis, TB or endocarditis, aneurysms or kidney stones? *Is the patient immunocompromised?*

Is there a **past history of structural deformity of your back?**

Have you slipped a disc in the past?

Do you suffer from osteoporosis?

Do you have a pacemaker implanted or have you ever had an intracranial aneurysm clipped? (Contraindications for a back MRI scan as part of the management plan)

➤ Drug history

Do you take any tablets or injections such as anti-inflammatory drugs or **steroids**?

Does the pain respond to analgesics?

Do you take HRT? (Osteoprotection)

➤ Social history (Yellow flags)

Do you **smoke?** How much and for how long? When did you stop?

How much **alcohol** do you drink?

Do you use recreational drugs? Please do not be concerned by me asking you the next question as I ask this to everyone presenting with a problem such as yours. **Do you suffer from HIV?**

Ask about overseas travel history, tropical illnesses.

What is your occupation? Does it involve manual work? What effect does your job have on the back pain and vice versa?

Back pain

Ask about exercise capacity, lifestyle limitations due to disease. Is driving a part of your job?

Have you taken time off work? How much? Why? What are the physical demands of your job? (Work characteristics) Do you enjoy your job? (Degree of job satisfaction) Are there any other health problems causing time off work? What are the conditions like at work? What is the social policy at your work place regarding taking time off for ill-health?

Are there any non-health problems, or problems unrelated to your current state of health, causing time off work?

Depression/psychiatric distress/illness behaviour? How is your mood? How are you coping at the moment?

What is the family's attitude and belief regarding the problem? (*Is there any evidence of reinforcement of disability behaviour?*)

Ask about personal problems – alcohol, family/marital, financial.

Are you participating in social activities? Does the pain interfere with hobbies?

How far can you usually walk, and what stops you?

How do the symptoms affect your sleep?

➤ Family history

Is there a family history of back conditions and malignancy?

Is there a family history of ankylosing spondylitis/psoriasis/IBD?

➤ Systemic enquiry

Especially musculoskeletal and neurology.

➤ Differential diagnosis

Mechanical back pain

- **Intervertebral disc prolapse**
- **Spinal stenosis (claudication-type pain)**
- Spondylolisthesis
- Spondylosis
- Trauma
- Non-specific back pain

Inflammatory back pain

- RA
- Seronegative spondyloarthritides
  - Psoriatic
  - Ankylosing spondylitis
  - Reiter's/reactive arthritis
  - Enteropathic (UC/Crohn's disease)
  - Behçet's

Referred pain

- **Aortic aneurysm/dissection**
- Pyelonephritis/renal calculus
- Acute pancreatitis/pancreatic carcinoma
- Penetrating peptic ulcer

'Sinister' back pain

- **Infection**
  - Discitis/osteomyelitis
  - Epidural/spinal abscess
- **Malignancy** (especially secondaries – breast, bronchus, thyroid, kidney and prostate)
- **Multiple myeloma**
- Osteoporotic crush fracture
- Paget's disease

➤ Investigations

Blood tests
- Haematology – FBC, ESR, blood film, cross-match/G+S
  - Anaemia (malignancy)
  - Raised WCC (infection)
  - ESR (malignancy, infection, inflammation)
  - Serum immuno-electrophoresis (myeloma)
  - Blood film (malignancy)
  - Cross-match/G+S (ruptured AAA)
- Biochemistry
  - U+Es (renal function)
  - Ca^{2+} (malignancy, myeloma, osteomalacia)
  - CRP (collections)
  - LFTs (malignancy, Paget's)
  - PSA (carcinoma prostate)
- Immunology
  - HLA-B27 status
  - Rheumatoid factor

Microbiology
- Blood cultures (sepsis)
- AAFBs (TB)

Urine
- Bence Jones proteinuria (myeloma)
- Blood, WCC (calculus, infection)

Radiology

- CXR
  - Metastases
  - Primary lung carcinoma
- Vertebral X-ray
- MRI back/spine
  - Degenerative changes
  - Spinal cord compression
  - Intervertebral disc prolapse
  - Osteolytic lesions
  - Space-occupying lesions (eg collections, metastases)
- Skeletal survey (myeloma)
  - Skull
  - Pelvis
  - Long bones (femurs)
  - Vertebral
  - Chest (ribs)

Further investigations

- Bone marrow aspirate/trephine (myeloma)
- Bone scan (malignancy, infection)
- USS (renal source, AAA)

Breast lump

➤ History of presenting complaint

Site

Where is the lump?

Onset

When did you notice it? (Duration)

How was it noticed? (Suddenly appeared, pain, itch, bleeding, change in pigmentation)

Character

How big is the lump?

Is it enlarging/staying the same/getting smaller?

Over what time course?

Has it changed in character over time? How?

Radiation

Have you noticed any other lumps similar to this one?

What about high in the armpit?

Associated symptoms

Is it producing any local symptoms?

Is there any nipple discharge/bleeding – from one or both nipples, one duct or multiple ducts?

Are there any skin changes – eczema, ulceration, retraction, discoloration/pigmentation, tethering, itching?

Are there any nipple changes – inversion, puckering etc?

Is it painful or causing discomfort?

Is there any heat/redness?

Ask about other symptoms suggestive of metastatic disease (bony, brain, liver, lung metastases, paraneoplastic syndrome):

- Swollen glands
- Fever
- Other lumps
- Weight loss
- Back/bone pain
- Breathlessness
- Jaundice
- Headaches
- Visual changes
- Fits
- Swollen arms
- Anorexia
- Changes in personality
- Tiredness

Precipitating factors

Is there any variation with the menstrual cycle, or throughout the month?

What do you think is wrong?

What are your concerns/ideas/expectations?

Ask about treatment, if any, already received.

➤ Past medical history

Is there any history of previous/serious illnesses or breast lumps/breast cancer?

Any previous treatments: mastectomies, wide local excision, radiotherapy, chemotherapy, breast reconstruction, other operations.

Have you suffered from breast disease in the past?

Have you had mammograms in the past? What were the results?

Is there a history of cancer in the other breast? Is there a history of cancer of the womb?

Is there a history of carcinoma ovaries/bowel? (BRCA1/BRCA2)

Pregnancy history

How many children do you have and how old are they?

Did you breast-feed your children? All of them? Were there any problems?

Gynaecological history

When did you start your periods?

When did your periods stop? What is your menopausal status?

Is there any history of previous gynaecological operations?

Have you had radiotherapy, eg for previous Hodgkin's?

➤ Drug history

Do you take any medications, including oestrogens or tamoxifen?

Have you had chemotherapy?

Have you ever been on the oral contraceptive pill or HRT and for how long?

➤ Social history

Ask about smoking and alcohol consumption.

➤ Family history

Is there a family history of malignancy – breast or ovarian cancers?

➤ Differential diagnosis

Non-breast lumps

- Lipoma
- Sebaceous cyst
- Retromammary abscess from chest disease (eg chronic empyema)
- Tietze's syndrome (costochondritis)
- Rib deformities
- Chondroma of the costal cartilages
- Mondor's disease (thrombosis of superficial veins of chest wall)
- Eroding aortic aneurysm

Generalised swelling

- Pregnancy
- Lactation
- Puberty
- Mastitis

Discrete breast lumps

Benign

- Fibroadenoma*
- Simple cyst*
- Fibrocystic disease*
- Abscess
- Fat necrosis
- Galactocele
- Duct ectasia
- Duct papilloma

Malignant

- **Carcinoma of the breast***
- Phylloides tumour/cystosarcoma phylloides
- Sarcoma/lymphoma

* Around 95% of all breast lumps are caused by one of these four conditions.

➤ Investigations

Blood tests

- Haematology – FBC, ESR
  - Anaemia (anaemia of chronic disease)
  - Raised WCC (abscess)
  - ESR (infection, malignancy)
- Biochemistry
  - CRP (infection)
  - LFTs (metastases)
  - Ca^{2+} (metastases)

Microbiology

- M,C+S (nipple discharge)

Radiology

- USS breast (best for young women/dense breasts)
- Mammography
- CXR
- Liver USS
- CT chest/abdomen/pelvis/brain
- Bone scan (if suspected breast carcinoma, for staging)

Pathology

- Fine-needle aspiration of breast lump
  - M,C+S
  - Cytology
- Core (Trucut) biopsy
  - Staging
  - Grading
  - Type of tumour (ductal, lobular etc)
  - Oestrogen receptor status
  - Lymph node involvement

Further investigations

- Open excision biopsy

Change in bowel habit

➤ History of presenting complaint

Onset

When did it start?

Timecourse?

Was onset sudden or chronic?

Frequency of defecation?

Character

What does the patient actually mean by a change in bowel habit?

What have you noticed:

- Increased frequency?
- Change in stool colour?
- Consistency of motion – well formed, watery, floating in the pan, smelly stools?
- Clarify what is normal for them?

Associated symptoms

Are there any other symptoms such as diarrhoea, vomiting or flushing?

malignancy, malabsorption –

- blood
- vomiting
- weight loss
- abdominal mass
- fever
- pain on defecation
- jaundice
- anaemia
- steatorrhoea
- mucus/pus
- tenesmus

Precipitating factors

Is there any clear precipitation by particular foods, travel, medication changes etc?

Relieving factors

medications eg. loperamide?

Severity

how is day-to-day living affected?

What do you think is wrong?

Ask about treatment already received?

➤ Past medical history

Is there a history of GI disorders, eg IBD, bowel malignancy, thyroid dysfunction?

Have you had previous abdominal surgery?

Have you had previous episodes of bowel obstruction due to, for eg adhesions?

➤ Drug history

Think about drugs which may have precipitated change.

➤ Social history

Overseas travel history, tropical illnesses.

Vaccinations (eg typhoid, hepatitis).

➤ Family history

Is there a FHx of IBD or gut malignancy?

> Differential diagnosis

Most commonly due to colonic disease. Possible causes include:

- **Neoplasia**
  - **Carcinoma of the colon, rectum or anus**
  - **Polyps**
- **Inflammation**
  - **Diverticular disease**
  - **Inflammatory bowel disease (ulcerative colitis, Crohn's)**
- **Ischaemia**
  - **Mesenteric thrombosis**
- **Irritable bowel syndrome (a diagnosis of exclusion)**
- Dietary change (fibre)
- Drugs – codeine, laxatives, iron, antibiotics

See also chapters on Diarrhoea and Constipation

> Investigations

Blood tests

- Haematology – FBC, ESR
  - Anaemia (carcinoma, IBD)
  - Raised WCC (infectious diarrhoea)
  - ESR (infection, inflammation, malignancy)
- Biochemistry
  - U+Es (dehydration if diarrhoea severe)
  - CRP (infection)
  - LFTs (IBD, metastases)
  - Ca^{2+} (metastatic spread to liver)

Microbiology

- Stool culture (infections)
- *Clostridium difficile* toxin assay

Pathology

- Biopsy on sigmoidoscopy/colonoscopy (carcinoma/IBD)

Radiology

- AXR (IBD)
- Barium enema (carcinoma, diverticular, IBD)
- Sigmoidoscopy/colonoscopy
- Small bowel enema/follow through (Crohn's)

Further investigations

- Angiography (mesenteric ischaemia)
- Staging CT (malignancy)

Chest pain

➤ History of presenting complaint

When did the pain start?

What were you doing when the pain started?

Were you well before the pain commenced? (Vomiting **before** the pain came on suggests oesophageal rupture; nausea and vomiting **after** the pain commenced suggests MI)

Have you had it before? If so, how was it different?

SOCRATES

Site

Did the pain go across your upper chest or upper abdomen? (Epigastric/sternal)

Onset

How quickly did it come on to reach a peak? (Instantaneous, seconds, over minutes, hours)

What was the duration of the pain?

Character

What does the pain feel like? (Tightness, gripping, pressing, crushing, like a weight, sharp, stabbing, like a knife, burning)

Is it constant or intermittent?

Radiation

Does the pain radiate anywhere? (To the arm, back, throat, jaw, teeth/gums, abdomen, along course of aorta and its branches)

Associated symptoms

Are there any other symptoms? Ask about:

- Nausea/vomiting
- Sweating
- Breathlessness (paroxysmal nocturnal dyspnoea, orthopnoea, on minimal exertion). What came first, the breathlessness or chest pain?
- Ankle swelling
- Palpitations (provocation, onset, duration, speed and rhythm of each episode, as well as frequency of episodes)
- Fever, rigors
- Anxiety

In this episode or on other occasions, did you ever feel like you're about to faint or indeed did faint? What stopped you fainting? (Dizziness, feeling of faintness, pre syncope/syncope/collapse. NB: Aortic stenosis can cause exertional syncope)

Ask about:

- Acid reflux, waterbrash
- Abdominal pain, neck pain/tenderness, leg pain
- Blurring of vision (aortic dissection)
- Cough, haemoptysis (PE), wheeze, purulent sputum

Has there been any recent viral illness/chest infection?

Precipitating factors

Is the pain precipitated by anything? (Cold, exercise/exertion, anxiety/ emotion, inspiration/breathing, coughing, movement (especially of trunk and arms, makes a musculoskeletal cause more likely), posture/ bending over/stooping, food, lying flat, heavy lifting, tight clothes, hot drinks, alcohol, swallowing)

What brings it on/what made the pain worse?

Does breathing affect the pain? (Pleuritic chest pain)

What about breathing deeply? Did movement or coughing make the pain worse?

Is the pain site tender when you press on it?

Relieving factors

What took the pain away? (Swallowing, belching, rest, posture (leaning forward), nitrates/GTN, oxygen, analgesia, antacids, cold drinks (hot drinks exacerbate GORD, cold drinks make it better))

How long did it take? (GTN relieves the pain of oesophageal spasm more slowly than cardiac chest pain)

Severity

Is it the worst pain you have ever had? Score out 10.

Does it keep you awake at night for example?

Does it stop activity?

> ➤ *Cardiovascular risk factors*
>
> Modifiable – smoking; hypertension; DM; high cholesterol
> Non-modifiable – previous IHD/cerebrovascular disease/peripheral vascular disease; positive family history; age; sex

> ➤ *DVT/PE risk factors*
>
> Calf swelling/pain/redness/heat, previous PEs/DVTs, recent travel, immobility, surgery, family history of DVTs/PEs, pregnancy, malignancy
> Have you coughed up any blood? (PE)

Muscular injury

Is there a history of trauma/injury/heavy lifting preceding the event?

Pericarditis

Is there any history of recent viral-like illnesses?

Other

Ask about contraindications to thrombolysis – active bleeding, previous haemorrhagic stroke, severe high BP, recent trauma/surgery, warfarin, recent head injury, known peptic ulcer, any bleeding tendencies, previous allergic reaction to thrombolytics, previous administration of streptokinase, pregnancy.

What do you think is wrong?

Have you received any treatments? (Aspirin, GTN etc)

➤ Past medical history

MITJTHREADS

Are you diabetic?

Were you born with any heart problems? (Septal defects)

Is there a history of IHD, angina, MI, intermittent claudication?

Have you had any cardiac operations (ballooning, bypass)?

Have you had any recent dental work (infective endocarditis)?

Do you have any known heart murmurs, prosthetic valves or pacemakers in place?

Is there a history of pulmonary disease (eg reversible airways obstruction and implications for future use of β-blockers; chest tightness may be a feature of COPD/asthma; past history of PE, pneumothorax)

Do you suffer from dyspepsia/hiatus hernia/dysphagia? Have you had a recent endoscopy?

Is there history of any recent instrumentation? (Oesophageal rupture/ pneumothorax)

Have you ever had shingles?

➤ Drug history

Do you take any tablets or injections, such as aspirin, warfarin or GTN spray?

Are you on tablets for hypertension or high cholesterol?

Have you ever had streptokinase, or do you carry a card saying you have had it previously?

Have you had a recent course of antibiotics? (Infective endocarditis)

Compliance, side-effect(s) of medication, OTC/herbal remedies, allergies.

(What happens?)

➤ Social history

Do you smoke? How much? For how long? When did you stop? (Ask if they have tried to stop, or congratulate them for stopping)

Ask about alcohol intake.

Do you use recreational drugs? (Infective endocarditis, cocaine and coronary vasospasm)

What is your exercise capacity? (Lifestyle limitations due to disease)

Does angina interfere with your life/work? In what way?

What is your occupation? (And its exposures)

Is driving a part of your job? If so, do you have a HGV/PSV licence? (Find out what effect cardiac conditions may have on occupation)

How far can you usually walk, and what stops you?

How do the symptoms interfere with your life? (Working, sleeping)

➤ Family history

Are your parents alive and well? *Is there a family history of IHD, hyperlipidaemia, sudden death, cardiomyopathy, congenital heart disease or Marfan's syndrome?*

➤ Differential diagnosis

Cardiovascular

- **Myocardial infarction**
- **Aortic dissection**
- Angina
- Pericarditis
- Aortic stenosis

Respiratory

- **Pneumothorax**
- **Pulmonary embolus**
- Pneumonia
- Pulmonary neoplasm

Gastroenterology

- Peptic ulcer
- Ruptured oesophagus (Boerhaave's syndrome)
- Oesophageal reflux
- Oesophageal spasm

Musculoskeletal

- Chest wall injury/fractured rib
- Costochondritis
- Herpes zoster (shingles)

> Investigations

Blood tests
- Haematology – FBC, clotting, D-dimers, ESR, cross-match/G+S
  - Anaemia (angina)
  - Raised WCC (pneumonia)
  - Clotting (dissection)
  - D-dimers (PE)
  - ESR (coronary vasculitis)
  - Cross-match/G+S (dissection)
- Biochemistry
  - U+Es (renal function, arrhythmias)
  - Ca^{2+}, magnesium (arrhythmias)
  - TFTs (hyperthyroidism → angina; hypothyroidism → raised cholesterol)
  - Glucose (modifiable risk factor)
  - Lipids (modifiable risk factor)
  - CRP (infection)
  - LFTs (cardiac cirrhosis)
  - Cardiac enzymes – troponin I/T (MI)

Microbiology
- Blood cultures (infective endocarditis, pneumonia)

Arterial blood gases (PE, pneumonia)

ECG
- Angina, non-ST-elevation MI, ST-elevation MI
- Arrhythmia
- Pericarditis

Urine dipstick
- Glucose (DM)
- Blood (infective endocarditis)

Radiology

- CXR
  - Large heart (cardiac failure)
  - Consolidation
  - Pneumothorax
  - Dissection (widened mediastinum)
  - Oesophageal rupture (pneumomediastinum)
  - Neoplasm
- CT with contrast (dissection)
- Aortography (dissection)
- V/Q scan or CTPA (pulmonary embolus)
- Echocardiography (transthoracic or transoesophageal)
  - Valvular dysfunction
  - Pericardial effusion
  - Vegetations (infective endocarditis)
  - Residual LV function and ejection fraction
  - Left ventricular hypertrophy
  - Pulmonary hypertension (PE)

Further investigations

- USS (gallstones)
- OGD (oesophagitis, peptic ulcer)
- 24-hour pH studies (oesophagitis)
- Oesophageal manometry (oesophageal spasm)
- Spirometry
  - Reversible airways obstruction and implications for use of β-blockers
  - Chest tightness may be a feature of COPD/asthma
- Ambulatory ECG monitoring
- Exercise tolerance test (cardiac risk stratification)
- Stress echo – exercise or pharmacological (dobutamine, dipyridamole) – risk assessment and assessment of myocardial viability
- Cardiac angiography (definitive diagnosis of coronary artery disease)
- Nuclear cardiological techniques and myocardial perfusion imaging (eg MUGA scan, SPECT, hibernation scans, functional MRI)

Collapse, syncope and blackouts

The history of the collapsed patient requires a collaborative/corroborative history from the patient, relatives, witnesses and ambulance officers.

➤ History of presenting complaint

Distinguish **syncope** (sudden, brief LOC with loss of postural tone and spontaneous recovery) from **dizziness/pre-syncope** (without LOC and postural tone) and **vertigo** (sensation of movement of themselves or the surroundings). Vertigo is covered in a separate section.

Consciousness – Did the patient lose consciousness, or not?

When and where did the patient collapse?

What was the patient doing at the time? (Standing, sitting, lying down, talking mid-sentence, turning head, exercising, sleeping etc)

Prior to episode

How did they feel immediately prior to the episode?

Was there any chest pain?

Was there any warning or prodrome? (Cardiovascular or neurological, eg distant, quiet voices, flushing, sweating, aura, blurring of vision, 'legs turning to jelly', automatisms – smacking lips, sinking/rising feeling in stomach, *déjà vu*, *jamais vu*, tastes, smells). Did the patient have time to warn bystanders/witnesses before they went down?

Associated symptoms

Was there any nausea, vomiting, sweating, headache, photophobia, neck stiffness, vertigo, palpitations, chest pain, breathlessness, pins and needles in the fingers/around the mouth? Did the patient feel sleepy (narcolepsy) before the attack?

Did it follow standing from sitting, prolonged standing, vigorous coughing, or occur during micturition/swallowing/defecation, head turning, nausea?

Precipitating factors

For example, being in a hot room, heavy meal, dehydration, sight of blood, emotion, fear, pain, watching a disturbing film, standing, pain, exercise, hyperventilation, turning head to the side, reaching up to the top shelf, neck movements, shaving, wearing a tight collar, stroboscopic lights/watching TV, sleep deprivation.

Was the patient limp or stiff when they fell to the ground?

Did someone try to hold the patient to prevent them from falling?

Did their eyes roll back?

During the episode

How long did the episode last? (Seizures last minutes, syncope rarely lasts > 60 seconds)

Were you unconscious? For how long? How long did any fitting last? (A good memory of events during episode suggests no LOC.) If there was no LOC, was the patient actually aware of what was going on? (Simple vs complex partial seizure)

Do you recall the falling process? How long were you on the ground? Do you remember this?

Are there signs of injury occurring during the collapse? Did they hit their head on the way down? (Suggests no warning and often LOC).

Were there any convulsive/jerking movements? Was it symmetrical/asymmetrical?

Was there any tongue-biting, urinary/faecal incontinence, frothing at the mouth? Did they bite the front or side of their tongue? Was the tongue macerated afterwards?

Was there a cry (may occur in tonic phase of a fit)?

Were there any focal features at the onset? (Sustained deviation of head or eyes or unilateral jerking of the limbs?) Where did it start?

What colour was the patient during and after the attack? Pale (deathly pale in Stokes–Adams), flushed, blue, grey, sweating? Ask witness.

What was the patient's breathing like during the episode?

Did the witness manage to take the patient's pulse during the episode? Was it palpable? (Slow in vasovagal attacks and AV block) Are they able to tap out the rhythm?

After the episode

Can he witness tell how long it took the patient to recover?

How did you feel afterwards? Were you confused, amnesic or tired/drowsy? Were your muscles aching? Did you have a headache or did you vomit? (Air insufflation of stomach in seizure) Was there any weakness of any limb(s) afterwards (to a lesser, greater, or similar extent compared with during fall; how long did this continue for?) Were you able to continue conversation afterwards?

Any symptoms suggesting blood loss? (Concealed/covert haemorrhage – weakness, postural dizziness, thirst, dry mouth, oliguria, feeling cold, shivering, breathlessness and altered mental status, eg leaking AAA)

What colour were you afterwards? (Flushed – suggestive of cardiac arrhythmia, pale, cyanotic, sweaty, warm (seizure) or cold (syncope))

Did you manage to get up independently, or did you need assistance? Were you able to resume activity straight away?

Was there a need for hospitalisation afterwards, for investigation and treatment with sedation or intravenous fluids, for example?

Were there any other symptoms, eg nausea, sweating, palpitations, chest/back pain, breathlessness?

Cardiovascular risk factors – see Chest pain.

DVT/PE risk factors and prior calf swelling? (Haemoptysis – PE, see Shortness of breath)

Were there any symptoms suggestive of a hypoglycaemic episode – hunger, jittery, faints, palpitations, sweaty, headache, confusion, coma?

Any previous episodes should be similarly analysed in detail.

What do you think is wrong? What are your concerns? (Losing your driving licence?)

Ask about treatment, if any, already received.

➤ Past medical history

MITJTHREADS

Have you had any previous falls? What were the circumstances?

Are you diabetic and on insulin? (Risk of hypoglycaemia leading to syncope) Healthcare worker with access to insulin?

Is there any history of previous cardiovascular disease, neurological disease, epilepsy, strokes, COPD, enlarged prostate, head injuries?

Do you have a pacemaker? When was it last tested?

Do you have a history of epilepsy? Febrile convulsions? Previous history of trauma? Sleep deprivation? Did you drink alcohol or misuse any substance prior to/the night before the episode?

Have you suffered from meningitis/encephalitis in the past? *Did they sustain injury at birth, or a period of perinatal hypoxia? Take a full developmental history, noting any specific insults.* (Epilepsy)

Have you ever had an EEG?

➤ Drug history

Do you take any tablets or injections?

Do you take any drugs that may cause hypotension, or predispose to falls (eg benzodiazepines/sedatives, antihypertensives, vasodilators – GTN, calcium-channel blockers, cardiac antiarrhythmic drugs, tricyclic antidepressants, dopaminergic medication)?

➤ Social history

Do you consume alcohol? Were you intoxicated at the time of the collapse? *Establish patient's alcohol history.* Does the collapse bear any relation to intake of alcohol?

Do you use recreational drugs? Have you overdosed in the past?

Assess how collapse at work would put patient's life at risk, as well as others, eg airline pilot, HGV driver. Do you currently drive?

Have you taken time off work? How much?

How do the symptoms interfere with your life? (Walking, working, sleeping)

➤ Family history

Is there a family history of sudden death, eg long-QT syndrome or cardiomyopathy?

Is there a family history of epilepsy?

➤ Systemic enquiry

Especially cardiology and neurology.

➤ Differential diagnosis

Cardiovascular

- **Orthostatic/postural hypotension** (drugs, hypovolaemia/haemorrhage, autonomic neuropathy, eg DM, Addison's)
- **Cardiac arrhythmia** (AV block/Stokes–Adams attack) including sick-sinus syndrome
- **Critical aortic stenosis**
- **Myocardial infarction**
- **Aortic dissection**
- **Vasovagal syncope**
- **Situational syncope** (micturition/post-prandial/cough/effort/swallowing/defecation)
- **Pulmonary embolism**
- **Shock** (haemorrhagic, septic, cardiogenic, anaphylactic, neurogenic)
- Carotid sinus hypersensitivity
- Hypertrophic obstructive cardiomyopathy (HOCM)

Neurology

- **Epilepsy/seizures**
- **Subarachnoid haemorrhage**
- Vertebrobasilar insufficiency
- TIA/stroke (rarely)
- Narcolepsy
- Subclavian steal

Metabolic

- **Hypoglycaemia**

Psychogenic

- Pseudoseizure
- Hyperventilation syndrome

➤ Investigations

BMs stat (glucose)

Blood tests

- Haematology – FBC, D-dimers
  - Anaemia (exacerbates syncope, bleeding causing collapse)
  - Raised WCC (sepsis)
  - D-dimers (PE)
- Biochemistry
  - U+Es, including Ca^{2+} and magnesium (precipitates arrhythmias, seizures)
  - Glucose (hypoglycaemia, seizures)
  - CRP (sepsis)
  - Cardiac enzymes – troponin I/T (cardiac event)
  - Prolactin (seizure)
- Arterial blood gases (PE, hypoxia causing seizure)

Microbiology

- Blood cultures (sepsis)

Urine

- M,C+S (UTI)

ECG

- MI
- Arrhythmia
- AV block
- LVH as evidence of aortic stenosis, HOCM
- 24-hour tape (paroxysmal arrhythmia)

Radiology

- CXR
  - Large heart (cardiac failure)
  - Dissection (widened mediastinum)
- Echocardiography
  - Aortic stenosis
  - HOCM
  - Right ventricular dilatation/hypertrophy (PE)
  - CCF (arrhythmias)
- CT head
  - Subarachnoid haemorrhage
  - Space-occupying lesion causing seizure (tumour, abscess, haematoma)
  - Haematoma from head injury sustained in fall
- V/Q scan or CTPA (pulmonary embolus)

Further investigations

- EEG (± sleep-deprived or ambulatory EEG) (epilepsy)
- Short SynACTHen test (Addison's disease)
- Implantable loop recorders/cardiomemo devices/Reveal devices (occasional arrhythmias)
- Tilt table test (vasomotor syncope)
- Carotid sinus massage (carotid sinus hypersensitivity)
- Carotid Doppler (carotid stenosis in recurrent TIAs)
- MRI brainstem (vertebrobasilar ischaemia)
- Lumbar puncture (subarachnoid haemorrhage, meningitis)
- Urine/plasma toxicology screen (drug overdose, seizure)

Confusion

Ask relatives/witnesses/friends/carers too in order to obtain a thorough history.

➤ History of presenting complaint

Onset

When did the patient first become confused?

How did it manifest?

How quickly did it come on? Was it recent or slow onset?

Character

Is there a difference in behaviour between night and day?

Does it fluctuate?

Does patient understand why they are in hospital?

Is patient 'up' or 'down' (delirium), or normal (dementia) in terms of psychomotor activity?

Are there any changes in memory?

Are they disorientated?

Is there a change in conscious level?

Does the patient have hallucinations, illusions or delusions? Are the hallucinations auditory or visual?

Associated symptoms

Is the patient's speech coherent?

What is their eyesight and hearing like?

Are there any other symptoms:

- UTI
  - Urinary frequency
  - Dysuria

- Incontinence
- Urgency
- Offensive smelling urine
- Sepsis (pneumonia/meningitis)
  - Fever
  - Headache
  - SOB
  - Cough
  - Purulent sputum
  - Chest pain
- Psychiatric illness
  - Depression
- Metabolic derangement
  - Thyroid disease: hyper/hypothyroidism

Precipitating factors

Are there any clear precipitants? eg changes in medication, recent operations, hospitalisations, alcohol withdrawal?

Have there been any recent falls, head injuries? (subdural)

What have the relatives, friends or other carers, including nurses noticed?

What was the **pre-morbid state** like compared with now?

Risk factors

Are there any risk factors for vascular disease? (See chapter on Chest pain)

What do they think is wrong?

Ask about treatment, if any, already received?

➤ Past medical history

Is there a history of previous episodes of confusion like this?

Are they diabetic and missing meals?

Have they had a previous stroke or MI?

Is there a history of significant physical or psychiatric illnesses?

Is there a history of Parkinson's disease?

Is there pre-existing dementia? Are they forgetful? Has their personality changed?

➤ Drug history

Gather a full drug history especially regarding:

- Sedatives
- Anticonvulsants
- Steroids
- Anticholinergics
- Opiates

Have there been any recent changes made to their medications?

➤ Social history

Alcohol intake. **Does the patient have a problem with alcohol dependence or withdrawal? What is their diet like and is vitamin deficiency possible?**

Have they used recreational drugs?

Living conditions at home? Risk assessment, eg boiling water, cooking/gas and heating? Family input?

Are other services involved? What are the attitudes, availability and willingness of others?

Establish the usual domestic arrangements, if there are any changes and the patient's usual functional abilities.

How do the symptoms interfere with their life (walking, working, sleeping)?

➤ Family history

Is there a FHx of Wilson's or Huntington's diseases?

➤ Systemic Enquiry

A full **functional enquiry** is vital as it may reveal symptoms of chest infection, subdural haematoma etc.

➤ Differential diagnosis

Intracranial

Infection

- Meningitis
- Encephalitis
- Abscess
- Subdural empyema
- Cerebral malaria

Vascular

- Infarct (TIA/stroke)
- Haemorrhage (especially subdural haematoma)
- Space-occupying lesion
- Venous thrombosis
- Vasculitis
- Malignant hypertension

Epilepsy

- Status epilepticus
- Complex partial seizure
- Post-ictal

Neoplasia

- Primary
- Secondary/cerebral metastases

Trauma

- Concussion/haematoma

Confusion

Extracranial/systemic

Infection
- UTI (urosepsis)
- Pneumonia
- Septicaemia
- Surgical wound
- Intravenous lines

Hypoxia
- MI/cardiac failure
- Respiratory failure
- Pulmonary embolus
- Hypovolaemia/haemorrhage
- Anaemia

Drugs and alcohol
- Side-effect
- Intoxication
- Withdrawal

Pain and discomfort
- Any cause including urinary/faecal retention

Metabolic
- Renal failure
- Liver failure
- Deranged sodium/potassium
- Deranged calcium/magnesium
- Acid-base disturbances
- Thiamine (Wernicke-Korsakoff syndrome), nicotinic acid or B_{12} deficiency
- Hypothermia/hyperpyrexia

Endocrine
- Glucose (hypo/hyperglycaemia)
- Thyroxine (hypo/hyperthyroidism)
- Cortisol (Cushing's/Addison's)
- Parathyroid hormone (Ca^{2+})

Inflammatory
- SLE

Psychiatric

- Acute-on-chronic dementia

➤ Investigations

- BMs stat (glucose)
- Temperature
- Pulse oximetry (oxygen saturation)

Blood tests

Haematology – FBC, D-dimers, haematinics

- Anaemia
- MCV (alcohol, hypothyroidism, vitamin B_{12} deficiency)
- Raised WCC (infection, infarction)
- D-dimers (PE)
- Haematinics (vitamin B_{12} deficiency)

Biochemistry

- U+Es (dehydration, renal failure, electrolyte anomalies)
- Calcium
- TFTs (hypothyroidism)
- Blood glucose
- CRP (infection)
- LFTs (alcoholic liver disease, disseminated malignancy)
- Cardiac enzymes – Troponin I/T (MI)
- Digoxin levels (digoxin toxicity)

Microbiology

- Blood cultures (sepsis)
- Urine (MSU/CSU) (UTI)
- Sputum
- Wound swabs
- Intravenous catheter tips
- Syphilis (VDRL) / HIV serology

Arterial blood gas (PE, pneumonia, respiratory failure)

Confusion

Urine

- UTI
- DKA

ECG

- Silent MI
- Electrolyte disturbances
- Digoxin toxicity

Radiology

CXR

- Consolidation
- Pulmonary oedema

CT head

- Ischaemia
- Bleed
- Space-occupying lesion

V/Q scan or CTPA (pulmonary embolus)

Further investigations

- Plasma/urine toxicology screen (drug overdose/intoxication)
- EEG (epilepsy)
- Blood film (thick and thin) (malaria)
- Lumbar puncture (meningitis, encephalitis, NPH)

Constipation

➤ History of presenting complaint

What do you mean by constipation?

What is normal for you?

When were your bowels last open?

SOCRATES

Onset

How long have you been constipated?

Is it a recent or long-standing problem?

How often do you open your bowels each week?

Character

Do you have colicky abdominal pain?

Is there complete failure to pass flatus or faeces?

Is there any pain on passing faeces?

Is there pain around the back passage?

Has the shape of the stool changed, eg become pellet-like?

Associated symptoms

Is there any distension?

Is there any late vomiting?

Is there any abdominal pain? Is it relieved by defecation?

Is there any rectal bleeding?

Precipitating factors

Has there been any recent surgery/inflammation which may have caused a paralytic ileus?

Have you been on prolonged bed rest?

Are you dehydrated?

Do you have a low-fibre diet?

Has there been a recent change in your diet? (Because of generalised disease or because of admission to hospital with strange surroundings)

Have you reduced your food intake, or are you trying to lose weight and on a slimming diet?

Ask about features of:

- Myxoedema
  - Slow thinking
  - Menorrhagia
  - Weight gain
  - Coarse skin
  - Hair changes
  - Hoarse voice
  - Cold intolerance
- Hypercalcaemia
  - Nocturia
  - N+V
  - Mental disturbance
  - Abdominal pain
- Malignancy
  - Weight loss
  - Lethargy
- Psychiatric illness (anxiety or depression)
  - Change in sleep pattern, early-morning wakening, difficulty sleeping

Relieving factors

Lactulose, senna, Fybogel®, water, fruit and vegetables, high-fibre diet

Severity

How much time is spent straining at stool?

What do you think is wrong?

Ask about treatment, if any, already received.

➤ Past medical history

Is there any history of previous illnesses such as carcinoma of the bowel, diverticular disease, painful haemorrhoids?

Are you diabetic, or do you suffer from hypothyroidism?

Have you ever injured your spinal cord or had trauma?

Previous neurological conditions?

Do you suffer from IBS? (Alternating constipation and diarrhoea)

Have you had any recent bowel operations, or a haemorrhoidectomy?

➤ Drug history

Do you take any medications, such as opioids, atropine, or TCAs?

Have you abused laxatives in the past, causing an atonic bowel?

Have any changes been made to your tablets recently?

➤ Social history

Ask about:
- Alcohol intake
- Use of recreational drugs
- Overseas travel history, tropical illnesses
- Occupation (occupational exposures), stress

How do the symptoms interfere with your life?

Constipation

> Family history

Is there a family history of malignancy, Hirschsprung's or spina bifida?

> Differential diagnosis

Organic obstruction

(= mechanical causes of large-bowel and small-bowel obstruction)

- Adhesions
- Hernias
- Malignant strictures (carcinoma)
- Benign strictures – diverticular disease, Crohn's disease, UC
- Pelvic masses – fetus, fibroids, etc

Painful anal conditions

- Fissure-in-ano
- Prolapsed haemorrhoids
- Rectal prolapse

Adynamic bowel

- Aganglionoses – Hirschsprung's, Chagas'
- Senility
- Spinal cord injuries/disease/compression
- Hypothyroidism
- Biochemical disturbances – hypercalcaemia, hypokalaemia, uraemia
- Pseudo-obstruction
- Systemic sclerosis

Drugs

- Opioids
- Iron salts
- Anticholinergics (TCAs, phenothiazines)
- Chronic laxative abuse
- Aluminium-containing antacids

Constipation

Habit and diet

- **Dehydration**
- **Immobility and post-operative pain**
- **Low-fibre diet**
- Hospital environment
- Irritable bowel syndrome

Psychiatric

- Depression
- Anorexia nervosa

➤ Investigations

Blood tests

- Haematology – FBC, ESR
  - Anaemia (carcinoma, IBD)
  - Raised WCC (diverticulitis)
  - ESR (carcinoma)
- Biochemistry
  - U+Es (dehydration if obstruction)
  - Ca^{2+} (metastases, hypercalcaemia)
  - TFTs (hypothyroidism)
  - CRP (inflammation)
  - Glucose (diabetic autonomic neuropathy)
  - LFTs (metastases)

Urinalysis

- High specific gravity if fluid intake inadequate

Pathology

- Biopsy on colonoscopy (carcinoma/IBD/Hirschsprung's)

Radiology

- AXR (obstruction, megacolon)
- Barium enema (carcinoma, diverticular, IBD)
- Sigmoidoscopy/colonoscopy (tumour, diverticular disease, megacolon)
- USS (tumours, ovarian cysts, fibroids, pregnancy)
- MRI (spinal disease)

Further investigations

- Autoimmune profile (systemic sclerosis)
- CT scan (staging of malignancy, pelvic mass)
- Colonic transit studies
- Ano-rectal physiology

Cough

➤ History of presenting complaint

Onset

When did it start?

How long have you had the cough (chronic > 3 weeks) and how often does it happen?

Is there a history of choking and sudden onset? (Foreign body)

Character

Is it worse in the mornings (chronic bronchitis) or at night (LVF, asthma)? (Diurnal variation)

Is it affected by posture? (Bronchiectasis)

Is it progressive/continuous or variable/intermittent?

Do you get it every year/around the same time each year?

Character of cough:

- Barking (epiglottitis)
- Brassy (tracheal compression)
- Bovine or hollow (laryngeal nerve palsy)
- Immediately after eating/drinking (tracheo-oesophageal fistula, GORD, history of sinusitis)
- Night-time (asthma/CCF)

Is your cough effective/weak or poor at clearing secretions? (Bulbar palsy, expiratory muscle weakness)

Is the cough exacerbated by swallowing? (Aspiration)

Associated symptoms

Is it productive of sputum?

Ask about:

- Colour/quantity/quality/foul-tasting/odour
- Mucoid/purulent/bloodstained
    - Thin/serous/frothy – LVF (pink), hysterical (salivation)
    - Mucoid, grey/white/clear – chronic bronchitis
    - Mucoid, yellow – chronic bronchitis, asthma
    - Mucoid, green – bacterial infection, eg acute bronchitis, bronchiectasis, pneumonia, lung abscess
- Blood/haemoptysis?

Ask about:

- Fever
- Palpitations
- Pleuritic chest pain
- Weight loss
- Wheeze
- Stridor
- Breathlessness/difficulty breathing
- History of chronic respiratory disease? (COPD, bronchiectasis)

Ask about:

- Features of rhino-sinusitis (eg maxillary toothache, purulent nasal secretions/discharge, post-nasal drip, repeated throat clearing, excessive production of phlegm, facial pain)
- Features of CCF – shortness of breath/orthopnoea/PND, ankle swelling, palpitations
- Systemic features suggesting serious illness – weight loss, fever, night sweats, anorexia, immunosuppression

Precipitating factors

What triggers your cough?

- Home
- Holiday
- Work
- Seasonal variation
- Exercise

Does it occur every winter or is this a new symptom?

What time of day is it worst?

Have you had it for more than 3 months for two consecutive years? (Chronic bronchitis)

Risk factors for DVTs (Recent operations, immobility, long flights, long car journey) and calf swelling.

Do you suffer from heartburn, regurgitation or aspiration/previous infections? (*Is there any dyspepsia, reflux symptoms, or GORD?*)

Do you smoke?

Have you been exposed to particular infectious or chemical agents? (*Pertussis*, allergens, new medications such as ACE inhibitors)

Have you been in contact with others who are also coughing?

Have you ever had any trauma to the chest?

Relieving factors

Asthma inhalers?

Severity

Is it getting better, worse, or staying the same?

Have you fractured any ribs from the coughing, or has it ever been so bad that it has caused you to faint?

Or so severe that it caused urinary incontinence, worsening of bronchospasm or vomiting?

➤ Past medical history

Have you had any previous illnesses? (Asthma, heart failure)

Does your asthma inhaler help? (Usage, technique, number of times needed as rescue at work)

Is there a history of malignancy or TB? (Contact history in UK and India)

Travel/pets/household allergens? (Cats, dogs, pollens, dust mite, moulds, *Aspergillus* spores, etc)

➤ Drug history

Do you take any medications? (Especially ACE inhibitors and β-blockers)

➤ Social history

Do you smoke? How much and for how long? When did you stop? (Ask if they have tried to stop, or congratulate them for stopping)

Do you drink alcohol?

Use of recreational drugs?

Have you been abroad? (Overseas travel history, tropical illnesses)

Do you keep any animals at home?

Occupation (occupational exposures), exercise capacity, lifestyle limitations due to disease.

Have you taken time off work? How much?

How far can you usually walk? What stops you?

How do the symptoms interfere with your life (walking, working, **sleeping**)?

➤ Family history

Is there a family history of malignancy?

Have you been in contact with anyone with TB, or other infections?

❯ Differential diagnosis

Acute (≤ 3 weeks)

- **Foreign body**
- Infection
    - Upper respiratory tract infection (often viral)
    - Pneumonia
    - Infective exacerbation of COPD

Chronic (≥ 3 weeks)

- **Bronchial carcinoma**
- Infection
    - Pulmonary TB
- Pulmonary embolism
- Asthma
- COPD
- Congestive cardiac failure (cardiac asthma)
- Gastro-oesophageal reflux disease
- Rhino-sinusitis
- Bronchiectasis
- Diffuse parenchymal lung disease
- Drugs
    - ACE inhibitors
    - β-Blockers
- Chronic smoking
- Psychogenic

There are three main causes for a chronic persistent cough and a clear CXR:

- Asthma (50%)
- Rhino-sinusitis with a post-nasal drip (25%)
- Gastro-oesophageal reflux (20%)

Others (5%) include foreign body, bronchial adenoma, sarcoidosis, fibrosing alveolitis, ACE inhibitors.

> Investigations

Blood tests

- Haematology – FBC, D-dimers, ESR
  - Anaemia (malignancy, chronic disease)
  - Raised WCC (pneumonia), eosinophils (allergy)
  - D-dimers (PE)
  - ESR (malignancy, inflammation)
- Biochemistry
  - U+Es (renal function, SIADH in infection/neoplasia)
  - Ca^{2+} (malignancy, sarcoidosis)
  - CRP (infection)
  - LFTs (malignancy)
- Microbiology
  - Blood cultures (pneumonia)
  - Sputum M,C+S (including AAFBs)
  - Mantoux/Heaf test (TB)
- Arterial blood gases (PE, pneumonia)
- Peak flow (asthma)
- Pulmonary function tests
  - Spirometry
  - Reversibility (COPD vs asthma)
  - Flow–volume loops
  - Transfer factor

Radiology

- CXR
  - Consolidation (TB, pneumonia, COPD, sarcoidosis)
  - Aspiration
  - Bronchiectasis
  - Neoplasm
  - Inhaled foreign body
  - Cardiomegaly (cardiac asthma)
  - Fibrosis
- V/Q scan or CTPA (pulmonary embolus)
- (High-resolution) CT ± biopsy
  - Interstitial lung disease/fibrosis

- Bronchiectasis
- Diagnosis and staging of neoplasia

Further investigations

- Fibreoptic bronchoscopy (neoplasm, TB, bronchiectasis)
- Cytology (bronchial brushings, washings, BAL)
- Biopsy
- OGD (GORD)
- 24-hour oesophageal pH monitoring (GORD)
- Sweat test (cystic fibrosis)

Depression and anxiety

To begin with, I should like to get an idea of the sorts of problems that have been troubling you. What have the main difficulties been? Can you tell me more about that? Can you explain what you mean by . . . ?

➤ History of presenting complaint

How long have you been feeling like this for?

In what way has your mood changed (subjectively)/how do you feel generally in your spirits?

How would other people (friends and family) describe you (objective)?

How do they feel you have changed?

Do you feel tense, wound up or slowed down?

During the last month have you often been bothered by feeling down, depressed or hopeless?

During the last month have you often been bothered by having little interest or pleasure in doing things?

Do you still enjoy the things you used to enjoy (TV programmes/good book/radio/hobbies/sports/sex, etc)?

Have you lost interest in your appearance?

Can you still laugh and see the funny side of things?

Do you look forward with enjoyment to things?

Have you cried at all/felt tearful? How often?

Do you feel tired at all, lacking in energy or run down? Is there a reason why you should feel like this?

Are you still able to think about or concentrate on things the way you used to be able to (eg reading a book)? How is your level of 'get up and go'?

When in the day are you most low (diurnal mood variation)? What proportion of the day are you low? How is your sleep pattern? Do you experience early-morning waking? Do you suffer from lack of sleep/insomnia?

Do you ever feel like not getting up in the morning? Do you feel fresh in the morning after a good night's sleep?

Has your weight changed? How has your appetite been?

Exogenous vs endogenous trigger factors: Ask about jobs, school (exams etc), relationships, unemployment and days off work (beware of the sick role), financial problems, moving house, post-partum, someone close to them dying, health, chronic pain (eg post-shingles), chronic diseases (eg cancer, post-CVA, DM, epilepsy), alcohol misuse.

> ➤ *Risk factors for depression*

Previous depression

Lack of social support

Chronic physical disease

Unemployment

Positive FHx

Stressful life events

Suicide attempts

Alcohol/substance misuse

Post-partum

Are there any features of an **organic disorder** underlying the mood change such as:

- Hypothyroidism: weight gain, hirsutism, change in voice, skin changes, bowel function, heavy periods
- Cushing's: striae, thin skin, easy bruising, exogenous steroids, buffalo hump, moon face, acne, hypertension, obesity
- SLE: mouth ulcers, Raynaud's, photosensitive rash, joint pains
- Hyperthyroidism: weight loss, diarrhoea, eye changes, neck lumps, increased appetite, tremor, preference for cold weather, sweating

Depression and anxiety

Are there any features of **psychosis**?

➤ Hallucinations

Do you ever see things or hear noises/voices when there is no one else about/that other people around you don't appear to have seen or heard/that you can't explain?

Have you had any experiences recently that you've found difficult to explain? For example, some people tell me they hear voices when there is no one else around. Does that ever happen to you?

Does your imagination ever play tricks on you?

➤ Delusions

Do you ever believe you have any special powers?

Have you felt particularly concerned about your safety recently? Why?

Do you ever get the feeling that people are talking about you?

Have you felt lately that people are talking about you, plotting about you or trying to hurt you?

Does anything on TV/radio or in newspapers have any special meaning to you?

Has it ever appeared that any outside person is interfering with your thoughts in any way?

Do they put in or take away your thoughts?

Do you ever feel that other people can hear your thoughts?

Do you ever feel a person outside or an outside force is controlling your actions or feelings?

➤ Anxiety

Are there any features of anxiety-depression?

Can you sit with ease and feel relaxed?

Do you ever get a sort of frightened feeling like butterflies in the stomach, or as if something awful is about to happen?

Do you ever get sudden feelings of panic (chest pains, palpitations, hyperventilation, dizziness, tremor, pins and needles in fingers and around mouth)?

Do you ever deliberately go out of your way to avoid certain situations?

For mixed depression-anxiety, what seems worse – the depression or the anxiety?

Are there any features of obsessive-compulsive disorder: Do you find that you have to keep on checking things that you know you have already done? Do you spend a lot of time on personal cleanliness, like washing over and over, even though you know you are clean? Do you get worried at all by contamination with germs?

➤ *Mania*

Are there any features of mania (bipolar disorder)?

Have you ever had periods when your mood has been too high?

Have any of your friends or family said you have been a bit too high or irritable?

Have you sometimes felt particularly cheerful and on top of the world, without any reason?

Have you felt particularly full of energy lately or full of exciting ideas?

Do you feel restless, as if you have to be on the move?

Do things seem to be going too slowly for you? Have you developed new interests recently?

Are you easily distracted?

How has your sleep been?

Have you found you have needed less sleep than normal? Are you tired?

How has your sex drive been recently?

Have you spent a lot of money/gambled a lot recently?

Have you bought anything that you cannot really afford?

*In the **elderly** could this be dementia manifesting as depression (depressive pseudodementia)?*

Are they forgetful? Have you ever had any recent lapses in memory?

Risk assessment

Are they a danger to themselves (suicide/deliberate self-harm) or others?

Is there a history of mental illness?

What vulnerability factors are present?

See risk factors for depression (above) and suicide (below)

Suicidal intent

Have things ever got so bad that you have thought about harming yourself or others?

Have you ever felt like giving up or that your life is not worth living?

Do worrying thoughts ever go through your mind?

Have you ever acted on such thoughts (deliberate self-harm or suicide)? How often do these thoughts occur?

When was the last time you had such thoughts?

Are you scared of dying?

What are your thoughts about staying alive?

Have these thoughts ever included harming someone else as well as yourself?

Some women in this situation say they could not bear to leave their children behind without a mother and want to take them with them. Has this ever happened to you?

What do you hope to achieve by harming yourself and/or others?

What has stopped/saves you acting on such thoughts so far?

Have you made any definite plans? Have you told anyone?

What specifically have you thought about doing to yourself?

Have you taken any steps towards doing this, eg getting pills/buying a gun?

Have you thought about when and where you would do this?

Do you live alone? Have you made any attempts to avoid discovery? Have you made any plans for your possessions or left any instructions for people after your death, such as a note or will?

Have you thought about the effect your death would have upon family/friends?

What help could make it easier for you to cope with your problems at the moment?

How does talking about this make you feel?

Psychosocial factors – Beck's cognitive triad

How do you feel about yourself as a person (self), the world, the future? (Helpless? Hopeless? Worthlessness?)

Do you think you are a worthwhile person? Do you feel at all isolated? Are you currently unemployed?

Are there any solutions to your problems? Are you able to communicate at all with friends and family about how you are feeling?

> ➤ *Risk factors for suicide (SAD PERSONS)*

Sex (M > F)
Age (age > 40 but rising in young men)
DePression
Ethanol abuse
Rational thinking loss (especially psychosis)
Social support lacking
Organised plan
No pastimes
Sickness (medical disorders)

What do you think is wrong? (Does the patient have **insight** into their condition?)

Ask about treatment, if any, already received.

Depression and anxiety

❯ Past medical history

Ask about:

- Previous mental health illnesses.
- Psychiatric hospital admissions.
- Previous acts of deliberate self-harm/suicide? Did you seek any help afterwards?
- Childhood: health problems, education, school record, upbringing, parents, siblings.
- Personality: the patient's usual attitudes, moods, beliefs, interests, coping strategies.
- How would someone close to you have described you 3 years ago?
- Criminal offences?
- Traumatic events (abuse, assaults, serious accidents)?

❯ Drug history

Have you been prescribed any drugs?

What have you tried in the past? (Steroids (Cushing's), antidepressants, OCP, other psychotropic drugs; lithium, β-blockers (depression))

What is being actually taken?

Compliance, side-effect(s) of medication, OTC/herbal remedies, allergies. (What happens?)

❯ Social history

Do you smoke? How much?

Alcohol intake – **CAGE** questionnaire. (See page 7. **Two or more** positive replies identifies problem drinkers, **one** is an indication for further enquiry about the person's drinking.)

> May I ask you about your drinking habits?
> How much do you usually drink each day?
> Is alcohol in any way a problem for you? In what way?
> Have you had family problems because of drinking?
> Have you missed work because of drinking?
> Have you had morning shakes or other withdrawal symptoms?
> Have you had blackouts in the past from drinking?
> Have you heard voices or seen things in the past because of drinking?
> Have you had any drink-driving offences?

Use of recreational drugs:

- Have you ever experimented with any recreational/street drugs or substances of abuse?
- What route?
- How much do you spend?
- What effect does it have on your life?

Relationships, including children:

- *Number, duration, type, problems in family relationships?*

Sexual history:

- *Loss of libido?*
- *Loss of interest in sexual activity?*

Births, deaths and marriages.

Overseas travel history, tropical illnesses (antimalarials such as mefloquine (Larium®)).

Occupation: nature of work, problems at work. Taken time off work? How much?

Effect on social functioning. How do the symptoms interfere with life (walking, working, sleeping)?

➤ Family history

Is there a family history of suicide or depressive illness?

Depression and anxiety

> Systemic enquiry

Essentially to rule out **organic** disorders.

Have there been any other things lately that I have not covered?

> Differential diagnosis

Psychological causes of depression

- Adjustment reaction
- Bereavement disorder
- Dementia
- **Major depressive disorder**
- Dysthymic disorder
- **Bipolar affective disorder** (manic depression)
- Cyclothymic disorder
- **Alcohol- and substance-induced mood disorder**
- Psychotic depression (schizoaffective disorder)
- Mood disorder due to a general medical condition

Organic causes of depression

- **Hypothyroidism**
- Anaemia
- MS
- Malignancy
- **Drugs** – exogenous steroids, β-blockers, OCP
- **Cushing's syndrome**
- **SLE**
- Hypercalcaemia
- Depression associated with chronic disease – cancer, HIV etc
- Temporal lobe epilepsy (psychotic depression)

Psychological causes of anxiety disorders

- Normal response to a stressful situation, eg exams
- Phobic disorder
- Panic disorder
- Generalised anxiety disorder
- Obsessive-compulsive disorder
- Acute stress disorders
- Post-traumatic stress disorder

Organic causes of anxiety disorders

- **Drugs and alcohol intoxication/dependence/withdrawal**
- **Drug side-effect**
- **Hyperthyroidism**
- **Phaeochromocytoma**

➤ Investigations

Blood tests

- Haematology – FBC
  - Anaemia
- Biochemistry
  - U+Es, including Ca^{2+}
  - TFTs (hypothyroidism, hyperthyroidism)
  - LFTs (alcohol abuse)
  - Random/midnight plasma cortisol (Cushing's)
- Immunology
  - ANA, ENA (SLE)

Further investigations

- 24-hour urinary free cortisol (Cushing's)
- 24-hour urinary catecholamines (phaeochromocytoma)
- Dexamethasone suppression test (Cushing's)
- Urinary/plasma toxicology (drug overdose/intoxication)
- EEG (temporal lobe epilepsy)

Diabetes

➤ History of presenting complaint

Symptoms
- Polyuria
- Polydipsia
- Nocturia

DKA
- Polyuria
- Abdominal pain
- Breathlessness
- Drowsiness
- Polydipsia
- Confusion
- Changes in vision
- LOC

Complications of hyperglycaemia
- UTI
- Thrush (Candida)
- Fever
- Rigors (infection may precipitate deterioration)

Micro/macrovascular complications
- Chest pain
- Leg pain
- Numbness
- Paraesthesia
- Erectile dysfunction (impotence): Some patients with DM find it difficult to maintain erections. Do you have any problems like that?

Secondary causes of DM

- Cushing's
- Haemochromatosis
- Acromegaly
- Chronic pancreatitis

Is there also exocrine pancreatic insufficiency (malabsorption, weight loss, steatorrhoea)?

➤ Past medical history

Is there any history of known DM? How long have you had diabetes for?

What was the mode of presentation and what was the treatment?

Was it an incidental finding during blood/urine testing?

How is your glucose level monitored? (Frequency of urine testing, blood testing, HbA1$_c$, record books, awareness of hypos)

What has tightness of control been like?

How many emergency admissions have you had to hospital?

Ask about previous complications, if any.

Admissions for hyper/hypoglycaemia/DKA:

- Symptoms of hypoglycaemia – hunger, jittery, faints, palpitations, sweaty, headache, confusion, coma
- Symptoms of DKA – nausea, vomiting, hyperventilation, abdominal pain
- Do hypos ever occur at night?

Macrovascular complications

Vascular disease

- Heart disease – angina, MI, breathlessness (CCF)
- Stroke
- Peripheral vascular disease
    - Claudication
    - Leg/foot pain at rest
    - Ulcers

Foot care

Do you check your feet regularly? Do you visit a podiatrist?

Microvascular complications

- Peripheral neuropathy (numbness/tingling/pain)
- Autonomic neuropathy (vomiting, bloating, diarrhoea, gustatory sweating)
- Renal disease (proteinuria (frothy urine), microalbuminuria)
- Retinopathy (visual acuity, any laser treatments?)

Metabolic complications

- High cholesterol
- High lipids and hypertension – treatments?

Lifestyle

Diet/weight/exercise.

➤ Drug history

Full history of all diabetic therapy from time of diagnosis.

Are you taking any treatment for DM – diet alone, oral hypos, insulin (**what regimen**?)?

Ask about drugs that can be diabetogenic, eg corticosteroids, ciclosporin, thiazide diuretics

Are you taking β-blockers? (May cause hypoglycaemic unawareness)

Do you get lipodystrophy/atrophy/hypertrophy at injection sites? Do you vary injection sites?

Do you worry about gaining weight with insulin?

Are you happy with your regimen? That is, well controlled, but not too many hypos?

Compliance, side-effect(s) of medication, OTC/herbal remedies, allergies. (What happens?)

❯ Social history

Do you smoke? How much? For how long? When did you stop? (Ask if they have tried to stop, or congratulate them for stopping)

Ask about:

- Alcohol intake
- Exercise capacity, lifestyle limitations due to disease
- Interference with lifestyle

Who actually draws up the insulin/tests blood sugar, etc? (Patient/spouse/nurse)

Can you see to do it?

Have you taken time off work? How much?

How far can you usually walk and what stops you?

How do the symptoms interfere with your life (walking, working, sleeping)? Do you have hypos at night? Do you live alone?

❯ Family history

Is there a positive family history of diabetes mellitus, hypercholesterolaemia, micro/macrovascular disease, haemochromatosis etc?

Complications of diabetes mellitus

Heart

- **Accelerated atherosclerosis** (angina, MI, CCF)
- **Often cause of death**

Brain

- **Cerebrovascular disease** (TIAs, strokes)

Limbs

- Hands:
  - Cheiroarthropathy
  - Dupuytren's contracture
  - Carpal tunnel syndrome

Diabetes

- Small-muscle wasting
- Legs
  - **Peripheral vascular disease**
    - ➤ Ischaemia
  - Gangrene
  - **Ulceration**
    - ➤ Neuropathic
    - ➤ Ischaemic
    - ➤ Infective
- Clawing (→ pressure ulceration)
- Neuropathic arthropathy (Charcot's joints)

Eyes

- **Cataracts**
- Rubeosis irides
- Rubeotic glaucoma
- Infections
  - Conjunctivitis
  - Styes
  - Herpes zoster
- Diabetic maculopathy (type 2 > 1)
- **Diabetic retinopathy**
  - Background
  - Pre-proliferative
  - Proliferative (type 1 > 2)
- Oculomotor and other cranial nerve palsies (→ diplopia)
- Vitreous haemorrhage
- Retinal artery/vein occlusion
- Tractional retinal detachment

Kidneys

- **Diabetic nephropathy**
- Nephrotic syndrome
- Chronic renal failure
- Papillary necrosis
- Pyelonephritis, perinephric abscess
- Metformin-induced lactic acidosis

Diabetes

Nerves

- Symmetrical (mainly sensory) polyneuropathy ('glove and stocking' distribution)
- Acute painful neuropathy
- Asymmetrical (mainly motor) polyneuropathy (diabetic amyotrophy)
- Mononeuropathy
- Autonomic neuropathy
- Mononeuritis multiplex

Gastrointestinal

- Oral thrush (candidiasis)
- Gastroparesis
- Abdominal pain
- Vomiting
- Constipation
- Diarrhoea

Urogenital

- UTIs
- Polyuria
- Thrush/balanitis
- Erectile dysfunction

Rheumatological

- Joint stiffness
- Frozen shoulder
- Joint deformity

Dermatological

- Furunculosis
- Carbuncle
- Fungal infections
- Necrobiosis lipoidica diabeticorum
- Granuloma annulare
- Diabetic dermopathy

Sites of insulin injection

- Lipodystrophy
- Lipohypertrophy
- Lipoatrophy

Infections

Anywhere, but especially:

- Skin
- Gastrointestinal
- Urinary tract
- Lungs

Pregnancy

- Gestational diabetes
- Fetal macrosomia
- Obstetric and neonatal complications

Psychological (depression)

Associated with:

- Disease itself
- Disease complications
- Necessary lifestyle modifications
- Side-effect(s) of treatment

Other

- **Hypoglycaemic coma**
- Weight instability
- Brittle (uncontrolled) diabetes
- **Diabetic ketoacidosis**
- **Hyperosmolar non-ketotic coma**

➤ Investigations

There are four principal aims of investigations in the diabetic patient:

(i) to diagnose diabetes mellitus and assess level of glycaemic control

(ii) to determine trigger factors leading to poor glycaemic control (**i**nfection, **i**nfarction, **i**ntercurrent illness, **i**nsulin omission, **i**atrogenic (steroids))

(iii) to avoid the long-term complications associated with the condition

(iv) to exclude secondary causes of diabetes mellitus

Blood tests

- Haematology – FBC
  - Anaemia (chronic renal failure)
  - High WCC (infection)
- Biochemistry
  - U+Es (renal failure)
  - TFTs (associated autoimmune disease)
  - (Fasting) glucose (diagnosis)
  - Oral glucose tolerance test (if impaired glucose tolerance and for diagnosis)
  - Fasting lipids (modifiable risk factor)
  - HbA1$_c$ (accurate measure of glycaemic control)
  - Plasma osmolality (hyperosmolar non-ketotic)
  - Cardiac enzymes – troponin I/T (MI)

Microbiology

- Blood cultures (sepsis)

Arterial blood gases

- Metabolic acidosis (DKA)

ECG/exercise tolerance test/angiography (angina, MI)

Urinalysis

- Glucose (DM)
- Ketones (DKA)
- Proteinuria (renal failure)

Pus cells, organisms (UTI)

24-hour protein (microalbuminuria)/creatinine (diabetic nephropathy)

Radiology

- CXR (consolidation)

Further investigations

- Slit lamp examination ± tonometry (cataracts, glaucoma)
- Retinal photography and fluorescein angiography (diabetic retinopathy)
- Nerve conduction studies (peripheral neuropathy)
- Arterial Doppler USS/angiography (peripheral vascular and carotid disease)
- 24-hour urinary free cortisol/dexamethasone suppression test (Cushing's)
- IGF-1 (acromegaly)
- Amylase (pancreatitis)
- Serum ferritin (haemochromatosis)
- Sweat test/faecal elastase test (cystic fibrosis)
- 24-hour urinary catecholamines (phaeochromocytoma)

Diarrhoea

➤ History of presenting complaint

Onset

When did it start?

How quickly did it come on?

Duration

Have you had it before?

If so, how was it different?

When does it occur and how frequently?

How long does it last for?

Character

Try to establish what the patient actually means by the term 'diarrhoea':

Frequent stools?

Loose stools?

Liquid stools?

Loss of sphincter control – actually faecal incontinence?

Is there actually increased stool volume?

Is it extremely watery?

Is there undigested food in it?

Does it occur at night? (Organic vs functional)

Is there urgency/tenesmus? Incontinence?

What is the colour and consistency of the stool like?

Is the stool well formed?

Are there large or small volumes of stool?

Is any blood, mucus or pus present?

Diarrhoea

Are the stools pale, bulky, sticky, offensive, greasy? Do they float in the pan? Are they difficult to flush away? (Steatorrhoea)

If blood is present, is it mixed in, coating the surface of the stool, or only present on the toilet paper?

Is there usually some constipation, ie could this be spurious/overflow diarrhoea?

Associated symptoms

- Nausea/vomiting
- Abdominal pain
- Sweating/fever
- Rigors
- Jaundice
- Weight loss
- Skin rashes
- Arthralgia
- Back pain
- Mouth ulcers
- Eye changes

Symptoms of anaemia

- Fatigue, malaise, breathlessness, chest pain

Symptoms of fluid depletion

- Faintness, dizziness on standing up from sitting

How is the appetite? (Thyroid status)

Precipitating factors

What precipitated it?

Have you had any contact with others with diarrhoea and vomiting?

Have you been abroad and when? (Foreign travel history: country, city, rural; particular reference to timing of possible exposures, eg swimming in a particular river)

Have you eaten any 'dodgy' food recently?

- How long before symptoms started?
- What did you eat?
- Was it food or water?
- Where was it?
- Did you cook it yourself or were you in a restaurant?
- How was it cooked?
- Were fellow diners affected too, as far as you are aware?
- Is anyone else affected (either before or after you were)?
- Are you a vegetarian?

Dietary intake – especially wheat, rye, barley (and oats)?

Relieving factors

Ask about treatment already received, eg loperamide, antibiotics, antiemetics.

What effect did the medicines have on the diarrhoea?

Severity

Do you need to wear incontinence pads?

What do you think is wrong?

➤ Past medical history

Is there a history of previous diarrhoea or known GI disease, eg IBD?

Has there been growth retardation (malnutrition)?

Have you had any previous abdominal surgery? (Blind loops, short bowel, dumping syndrome)

Have you undergone radiation therapy? (Radiation enteritis)

➤ Drug history

Do you take any medications which may have precipitated the diarrhoea? (Laxatives, antibiotics (if within the last 3 months think of *Clostridium difficile*), NSAIDs, immunosuppressants etc)

Diarrhoea

> Social history

Do you consume much alcohol?

Sexual history – HIV-related diarrhoea (proctitis) etc.

Have you come into contact with TB?

Overseas travel history, tropical illnesses; vaccinations, eg typhoid, hepatitis.

> Family history

Is there a family history of IBD, gut malignancy, coeliac disease?

> Differential diagnosis

Infections

Gastroenteritis

- Bacterial
  - *Campylobacter*
  - *Escherichia coli*
  - *Salmonella*
  - *Shigella*
  - *Vibrio cholerae*
  - *Staphylococcus aureus*
- Viral
  - Viral enterocolitis, eg rotavirus
  - Astrovirus
  - HIV-related
- Parasitic
  - Amoebic dysentery
  - Giardiasis
  - Cryptosporidiosis

Inflammation

- **Inflammatory bowel disease (Crohn's disease, UC)**
- **Carcinoma bowel/villous adenoma**
- Diverticular disease
- Ischaemic colitis

Drugs

- Antibiotics (especially erythromycin)
- Alcohol
- Laxatives
- Magnesium-containing antacids

Malabsorption

- Short bowel syndrome, eg gastrectomy
- Bacterial overgrowth/blind loop syndrome
- Coeliac disease
- Pancreatic dysfunction
- Bile salts malabsorption
- Radiation enterocolitis

Endocrine

- Thyrotoxicosis
- Diabetes mellitus (autonomic neuropathy)
- Addison's disease
- Carcinoid syndrome
- VIPoma (Verner–Morrison syndrome)
- Zollinger–Ellison syndrome

Dysmotility

- Spurious diarrhoea (faecal impaction)
- Dietary
- Irritable bowel syndrome

Psychogenic

- Anxiety

Diarrhoea

> Investigations

Blood tests

- Haematology – FBC, ESR, haematinics, clotting
  - Anaemia (carcinoma, IBD)
  - Raised WCC (infectious diarrhoea, ischaemic colitis, IBD)
  - ↓ MCV (iron deficiency) or ↑ MCV (alcohol, coeliac, Crohn's)
  - ESR ↑ in carcinoma, Crohn's, UC
  - Iron and vitamin B_{12}/red cell folate ↓ in malabsorption
  - PT ↑ in reduced vitamin K absorption
- Biochemistry
  - U+Es (dehydration if diarrhoea severe)
  - CRP (infection, Crohn's, UC)
  - LFTs (IBD, metastases)
  - Albumin (malabsorption)
  - Ca^{2+}, phosphate (malabsorption)
  - Amylase (pancreatitis)
  - TFTs (hyperthyroidism)
  - Glucose (diabetic autonomic neuropathy, chronic pancreatitis)

Immunology

- Coeliac screen (antigliadin, antiendomysial, anti-tissue transglutaminase and antireticulin antibodies)

Microbiology

- Blood cultures (*Salmonella*)
- HIV serology
- Stool M,C+S X 3
  - Enterobacteria (*Shigella, Salmonella, Campylobacter, Escherichia coli*)
  - Virology (CMV, Norwalk, etc)
- Warm stool specimen for ova, cysts and parasites (eg *Giardia, Entamoeba histolytica*)
- *Clostridium difficile* toxin assay

Urinalysis

- Specific gravity high in dehydration
- Typhoid
- Urinary laxative screen

Pathology

Biopsies from OGD/sigmoidoscopy/colonoscopy (carcinoma/IBD/microscopic colitis/duodenal biopsy for coeliac disease/duodenal aspirate for giardiasis)

Radiology

- Abdominal film (IBD, toxic megacolon, pancreatic calcification)
- USS liver (liver metastases, carcinoid)
- Small-bowel enema/follow-through/enteroscopy (Crohn's)
- Barium enema (IBD, carcinoma, diverticular disease)

Rigid/flexible sigmoidoscopy (IBD, carcinoma, pseudomembranous colitis, villous adenoma)

Colonoscopy (tumours, colitis (extent and severity), diverticular disease)

ERCP ± pancreatic CT (pancreatic dysfunction)

Further investigations

- Angiography (mesenteric ischaemia)
- 24-hour urine collection for 5-HIAA and catecholamines (carcinoid, phaeochromocytoma)
- Serum gastrin (Zollinger–Ellison)
- Serum calcitonin (medullary carcinoma thyroid)
- Serum vasoactive intestinal peptide (VIPoma)
- Short synacthen test (Addison's)
- Faecal fat estimation (malabsorption)
- Hydrogen breath tests (hypolactasia (lactose) or small-bowel bacterial overgrowth (lactulose))
- 24-hour stool weights, repeated when fasting ('osmotic' vs 'secretory' diarrhoea)
- DEXA bone scan (osteomalacia secondary to vitamin D malabsorption)
- White cell scan (Crohn's)

Diarrhoea

- Other specialist pancreatic function tests:
  - Faecal elastase
  - Pancreolauryl test

Dizziness and vertigo

➤ History of presenting complaint

First try to establish what the patient actually means by the term.
Do they mean light-headedness, giddiness, unsteadiness
(disequilibrium), true vertigo (sensation of surroundings moving),
feeling faint (pre-syncope), headache, etc?

SOCRATES

Onset

When did it start?

Is it there all the time or does it come and go?

Are you dizzy at present?

How long does the episode last? (Minutes/hours/days)

How often are you dizzy/vertiginous? (Daily/monthly)

Was the onset sudden or gradual?

Have you had recurrent episodes or a single attack?

Is it intermittent or continuous?

Does it ever recover between episodes?

Does it terminate on its own?

Character

What does it feel like?

Associated symptoms

Is there any deafness (fluctuating or progressive) or tinnitus?

Is the deafness unilateral or bilateral?

Is there any discharge from the ear?

Is there any pain in the ear?

Is there any facial weakness or numbness?

Ask about:

- Headaches
- Nausea
- Vomiting
- Sweating
- Palpitations
- Chest pain

Are there any vesicles in or around the ear?

Is there a sense of fullness in one of both ears? (Hydrops)

Is there associated headache? (ICP, haematoma, acoustic neuroma)

Ask if there are any other symptoms suggesting a neurological cause, such as:

- Weakness
- Slurring of speech
- Visual disturbances
- Diplopia
- Dysphagia
- LOC
- Seizures
- Weakness
- Numbness/paraesthesia
- Clumsiness

Do you feel off-balance? Is there a tendency to fall to one side? (Are there any **cerebellar** symptoms – ataxia/gait disturbances, incoordination)

Are there any cardiovascular symptoms: chest pain (dizziness), palpitations?

Precipitating factors

Ask about:

- Trauma/head injury (labyrinth concussion, BPPV)
- Barotrauma/flying/swimming/diving (perilymphatic fistula)
- Head movement/position (carotid sinus hypersensitivity, vestibular pathology, vertebrobasilar insufficiency)
- Change in posture, rolling over in bed, exertion, etc

How long after changes in position do you get vertigo? Immediately implies central cause; after a few seconds' latency implies peripheral cause.

Are symptoms worse with the eyes open or closed?

Have you had any recent viral illnesses/ear infections that may have triggered the vertigo? (Vestibular neuronitis)

Do you have any limitation of neck movement? (Cervical vertigo)

Are you a migraine sufferer (or migraineur)?

Did any convulsions follow?

Is there anything else that may predispose the patient to falls – cataracts, proprioceptive loss, arthritides, foot problems, prosthetic joints?

Relieving factors

What alleviates the dizziness, eg sitting down, lying still?

Does it get better with repeated attempts at trying to elicit the vertigo? (That is, is it fatiguable, which implies a peripheral cause)

Does fixing your eyes on an object in the distance make any difference to the vertigo? What? (Peripheral causes of vertigo are suppressed by fixation)

Cardiovascular risk factors. See chapter on Chest pain.

What do you think is wrong?

Ask about treatment, if any, already received.

➤ Past medical history

Is there any previous history of serious cardiac or neurological disease?

Do you suffer from travel sickness?

Have you had previous episodes like this or of syncope/vertigo?

Do you suffer from migraines?

Do you suffer from epilepsy? (Epileptic vertigo)

Has there been concomitant or prior ear disease and/or ear surgery?

Have you had any recent viral illnesses, ear or sinus infections?

Has there been any recent head or neck trauma?

Do you suffer from panic attacks/anxiety?

➤ Drug history

Do you take any medications?

Have there been any recent changes to medications or an increase in doses?

Are you taking any drugs that might cause symptoms, eg diuretics causing postural hypotension, or phenytoin, gentamicin or furosemide causing vertigo?

Are you taking any treatments, eg vestibular 'sedatives' such as prochlorperazine, betahistine?

➤ Social history

Do you consume much alcohol? What effect does it have on the dizziness?

Do you use recreational drugs?

Have you been abroad? (Overseas travel history, tropical illnesses)

Accidental risk assessment at home, eg steepness of stairs?

Occupation (occupational exposures), exercise capacity, lifestyle limitations due to disease.

Have you taken time off work? How much?

Do you use walking sticks/aids? How far can you usually walk and what stops you?

How do the symptoms interfere with your life? (Walking, working, sleeping)

➤ Differential diagnosis

Dizziness/light-headedness

See Collapse/syncope. Commonly caused by:

- Orthostatic hypotension
- Cardiac arrhythmia
- Vasovagal syncope
- Situational syncope (cough, micturition, post-prandial)
- Carotid sinus hypersensitivity
- Anaemia
- Hypoglycaemia
- Anxiety (hyperventilation syndrome)

True vertigo (rotational)

Peripheral

- Vestibular
  - Ménière's disease
  - BPPV
  - Acute labyrinthitis (vestibular neuronitis)
  - Motion sickness
  - Trauma
  - Middle ear disease
  - Herpes zoster oticus (Ramsay–Hunt syndrome)
- Drugs and toxins
  - Aminoglycosides (eg gentamicin)
  - Furosemide
  - Quinine
  - Salicylate
  - Phenytoin
  - Alcohol intoxication

- Eyes
  - Ophthalmoplegia with diplopia
- Cervical vertigo

Central

- Brainstem and cerebellum
  - Demyelination (MS)
  - Ischaemia (vertebrobasilar)
  - Haemorrhage
  - Tumours
  - Basilar migraine (rare)
- Cerebellopontine angle
  - Acoustic neuroma (vestibular schwannoma)
- Cerebral cortex
  - Vertiginous (temporal lobe) epilepsy

➤ Investigations

Blood tests
- Haematology – FBC, vitamin B_{12} level
  - Anaemia (exacerbates dizziness)
  - MCV (alcoholism)
  - Vitamin B_{12} levels (vitamin B_{12} deficiency)
- Biochemistry
  - Glucose (hypoglycaemia)
  - LFTs (alcoholism)
  - Salicylate levels

Microbiology
- Gentamicin levels
- Syphilis serology

ECG
- Cardiac arrhythmia

Audiometry (if associated hearing loss)

Radiology

- CT
  - Haemorrhage
  - Space-occupying lesion
- MRI
  - Demyelination
  - Acoustic neuroma
  - Ischaemia
  - Space-occupying lesion
  - Posterior fossa/cerebellar lesions (eg cerebellar haemorrhage)

Further investigations

- Tilt table test (vasomotor syncope)
- EEG (temporal lobe epilepsy)
- Lumbar puncture (MS)
- Vestibular function tests including electronystagmography, calorimetry and brainstem evoked potentials

Double vision (diplopia)

➤ History of presenting complaint

Try to clarify what the patient means by double vision – is it really double vision or simply blurring of vision?

Do you wear contact lenses or glasses?

What is your prescription?

When was the last time you had your eyes tested?

Have you changed your glasses/contact lenses recently?

SOCRATES

Site

Is it unilateral or bilateral?

Onset

Was it gradual or sudden? (latter usually indicates a neurological cause)

Character

What happens when you cover one eye? Does the double vision disappear or does it persist? (monocular vs binocular diplopia)

If monocular, has the patient had previous corneal inflammation, or are there any features of a cataract (blurring of vision, increasing short-sightedness such that it allows the elderly patient to read without glasses (so called second-sight), glare especially when driving at night, haloes etc).

In which direction are the images furthest apart? Is it worse to the right/left/up or down?

Are the images separated vertically, horizontally or obliquely?

Is it worse for objects closer to or further away from you? (VI nerve palsy is worse for far, III nerve palsy worse for near)

What do you find difficult as a result of the double vision? (reading (loss of accommodation in III nerve palsy), eating, going downstairs? –implies IV nerve palsy). Have you found any ways of compensating (eg tilting your head to one side – IV nerve palsy)?

Is it all the time or intermittent? Is there any time of day when it is worst? (myasthenia). What about when your eyes are tired?

Have you noticed any other muscle weakness anywhere else in your body?

Have you noticed any changes to the pupil ('the black of your eye'), or eyelids, of either or both of your eyes? (III nerve palsy)

Associated symptoms

Is there any **eye pain**? (is it worse on eye movement) (optic neuritis, orbital myositis, intraocular SOLs, posterior communicating artery aneurysm)

Is there **blurring of vision**? (eg reading),

Are there **reduced visual fields**? (holes missing in the field),

Have you noticed a loss of **intensity of colours** such that everything looks grey or misty?

Is there nasal discharge? (NPC causing VI nerve palsy)

Are there any features of **hyperthyroidism** – eye changes/bulging eyes, weight loss, increased appetite, heat intolerance, diarrhoea, palpitations etc?

Are there any other neurological features that would indicate **meningitis, MS, brainstem infarct/tumour, raised ICP** (VI nerve palsy) – drowsiness, weakness, parasthesia/numbness, deafness, tinnitus, taste disturbances, bladder/bowel dysfunction, dysphagia, vomiting, headaches, photophobia, non-blanching rash etc?

Are there any fevers or chills? (meningitis, orbital/brain abscess, cavernous sinus thrombosis)

Precipitating factors

Is there a history of head injury/trauma, or blow out fractures?

What do you think is wrong?

Ask about treatment, if any, already received?

➤ Past medical history

Congenital eye abnormalities, such as amblyopia ex anopsia?

Have you had previous squints? Have you had squint surgery?

Are you diabetic?

Do you suffer from hypertension?

Do you have MS?

Have you had eye surgery?

Have you had TIAs/strokes or cranial neoplasms?

Have you sustained previous trauma to the eye? Have you had previous meningitis?

➤ Drug history

Do you take any medications?

Is there any evidence of intoxication – opiates, Benzodiazepines?

➤ Social history

Do you use recreational drugs? (intoxication)

Do you consume large amounts of alcohol? (intoxication)

Occupation (occupational exposures), exercise capacity, lifestyle limitations due to disease.

What is the extent of the visual disability?

Have you taken time off work? How much?

How far can you usually walk, what stops you?

How do the symptoms interfere with your life (walking, working, sleeping)?

Do you have adaptations at home to compensate?

Do you own a guide dog?

> Family history

Is there a FHx of Marfan's syndrome (ectopia lentis)?

> Differential diagnosis

Monocular

- Early cataract
- Corneal irregularity – Previous corneal inflammation/post-trauma
- True cortical polyopia (rare)
- Hysteria

Binocular

Congenital:

- Decompensated long-standing squint
- Duane's syndrome

Acquired:

- Central
  - **MS (internuclear ophthalmoplegia)**
  - Brainstem tumour/ischaemia (vertebrobasilar)
- Neurogenic (III, IV and VI Cranial nerve palsies)
  - **DM**
  - **Posterior communicating artery aneurysm**
  - Raised ICP (as a false localised sign or pseudotumour cerebri)
  - Intracranial SOL (tumour, haemorrhage, aneurysm, abscess, cavernous sinus thrombosis)
- Neuromuscular junction
  - **Myasthenia gravis**
  - Eaton–Lambert syndrome
- Myogenic
  - **Thyroid eye disease**
  - Orbital myositis
  - Intraocular space occupying lesion
  - Myopathies (oculopharyngeal muscular dystrophy)
- Other:
  - Refractive errors, incorrect spectacles

- Trauma (blow out fractures)
- Media opacities
- Drug and alcohol intoxication

➤ Investigations

Blood tests

- **Haematology : FBC, ESR**
  - Cerebrovascular disease
  - Inflammatory conditions
- **Biochemistry:**
  - **Fasting/random glucose** (diabetes mellitus)
  - **TFTs** (thyroid eye disease)
  - **Lipids** (cerebrovascular disease)
- **Immunology:**
  - **Anti-nAChR antibodies (myasthenia gravis)**

Urine

- **Glucose** (diabetes)

Radiology

- **Skull and facial bone X-rays** (blow-out fractures)
- **MRI/CT head**
  - Demyelination
  - Ischaemia
  - Head injury
  - Space occupying lesion
- **Angiography** (aneurysm)

Further investigations

- **Tensilon test** (myasthenia gravis)
- **EMG studies** (myasthenia gravis)
- **Lumbar puncture** (MS, meningitis)
- **Muscle biopsy** (myopathy)
- **Genetic studies** (muscular dystrophies)

Dyspepsia and indigestion

NB: Red flag symptoms as highlighted by the British Society of Gastroenterology are shown in **bold**. Presence of any (including age > 55 years) requires an urgent OGD to exclude carcinoma.

➤ History of presenting complaint

First establish what the patient actually means by dyspepsia (**abdominal pain**, dysphagia, reflux, retrosternal pain, bloating, nausea, etc).

SOCRATES

Site

Where do you feel it?

Is there bloating or fullness?

Onset

When did it start?

Character

What is the character of the pain or discomfort (eg burning, aching, stabbing)?

What does it feel like?

Radiation

Does the pain/discomfort radiate, eg to the back?

Associated symptoms

Is there any relation to exertion?

Consider a cardiac cause which can mimic dyspepsia.

Is there any:

- Waterbrash
- Acid brash
- Aspiration (with coughing)
- Bloating
- Nocturnal asthma
- **Anorexia** (due to pain or not?)
- **Early satiety**
- **Unintentional weight loss (> 3 kg) – carcinoma**
- **Odynophagia**
- **Dysphagia**
- **Jaundice**
- **Persistent vomiting**
- **Nausea**
- Change in bowel habit
- **Haematemesis**
- **Dark/black stools**
- **Any epigastric masses**
- **Symptoms of anaemia**
  - Fatigue
  - Angina
  - Breathlessness
  - Palpitations
  - Reduced exercise tolerance

Precipitating factors

When are the symptoms apparent?

After meals? After certain foods (spicy foods, coffee)?

After alcohol?

At night? Lying down?

During stooping? Heavy lifting?

When wearing tight clothes?

Relieving factors

Does anything relieve the symptoms?

- Sitting upright
- Antacids
- Drinking milk
- Bloating
- Belching

Severity

Is the pain severe enough to hospitalise the patient?

What do you think is wrong?

Ask about treatment already received.

➤ Past medical history

Is there a history of chest infections from aspiration, indigestion?

Has there been **previous peptic ulceration**?

Have you had previous endoscopies? What were the results?

Is there a history of treatment with PPIs or H_2 antagonists?

Is there a **history of stomach operations**, which increases the risk of gastric carcinoma (eg vagotomy and pyloroplasty causing biliary reflux)?

Is there any history of known gallstones (chronic cholecystitis)?

Have you had any barium meals in the past?

➤ Drug history

Do you take any medications, especially anti-inflammatories, warfarin, steroids, iron tablets (produces black stools), alcohol, codeine, co-proxamol, aspirin?

Do you take any treatments for dyspepsia (antacids, H_2 antagonists, PPIs)?

Have you ever taken a course of *Helicobacter pylori* eradication treatment?

➤ Social history

Do you **smoke**? How much and for how long? When did you stop?

Alcohol intake. (GORD, gastritis, PUD, varices)

How do the symptoms interfere with your life? (Walking, working, sleeping)

➤ Differential diagnosis

Oesophagus

- **Gastro-oesophageal reflux disease**
- Oesophagitis
- Oesophageal carcinoma

Stomach/duodenum

- **Peptic ulcer disease**
- Hiatus hernia
- Gastritis
- Duodenitis
- **Gastric carcinoma**

Gallbladder

- Chronic cholecystitis

Other

- Non-ulcer dyspepsia
- Chronic pancreatitis
- Pancreatic carcinoma
- Irritable bowel syndrome
- **Cardiac chest pain**

> Investigations

Blood tests
- Haematology – FBC, ESR
  - Anaemia (anaemia of chronic disease)
  - Raised WCC (infection/inflammation)
  - ESR (malignancy)
- Biochemistry
  - U+Es (renal function)
  - CRP (infection)
  - LFTs (gallstones, malignancy)

ECG (to exclude cardiac pathology)

Faecal occult blood (bleeding PUD, tumours)

OGD + biopsy for histology/*Helicobacter pylori* (tumour/PUD/Barrett's oesophagus/oesophago-gastritis)

Radiology
- Barium swallow (hiatus hernia, achalasia and other motility disorders, oesophageal tumours)
- Barium meal (PUD, gastric tumours)

Further investigations
- CXR (hiatus hernia)
- USS abdomen (gallstones/calcification of pancreas)
- CT abdomen (gallstones/chronic pancreatitis)
- Oesophageal pH studies (oesophageal reflux)

Dysphagia

➤ History of presenting complaint

Site

Where does the patient feel things are sticking? (Back of throat, suprasternal notch/top of neck, mid-sternum/bottom of chest)

Onset

When did it start?

How has this developed?

Is it progressive? (Weeks, months)

Character

Is there difficulty swallowing solids and/or liquids?

What about saliva – are you able to swallow it or do you drool at the mouth? (Total or absolute dysphagia)

Is it continuous or intermittent/variable?

Is it getting better, worse, or staying the same?

Can you eat a full meal?

Is it difficult to make a swallowing movement?

Associated symptoms

Is it painful when you swallow, or at any other times? (Odynophagia)

Is it the pain stopping you from swallowing, or does the food actually get stuck?

Is there bulging of the neck or gurgling, especially after meals/drinking fluids?

Do you get bad breath? (Halitosis)

Do you cough or suffer from asthma at night? (Nocturnal asthma)

Is there any coughing/choking with swallowing or lying down?

Is there any nasal regurgitation? (GORD or aspiration)

Is there any:

- Vomiting
- Nausea
- Regurgitation
- Haematemesis
- Weight loss
- Anorexia
- Jaundice
- Hoarse voice
- Associated heartburn/chest pain/abdominal pain?

Are there any symptoms of anaemia?

- Reduced exercise tolerance
- Fatigue
- Angina
- Breathlessness

Is there a change in bowel habit? Do you have dark/black stools?

Is there any evidence of weakness elsewhere?

Do you have mouth ulcers? Do you have good dentition? Are your dentures well fitted?

Is there a history of a foreign body, eg a fish bone getting stuck in the throat?

Are there any features to suggest scleroderma – skin changes, Raynaud's/ cold hands, changes in face, arthritis, etc

Precipitating factors

Is there chest pain between meals? (PUD)

Or while swallowing? (Oesophagitis)

Has there been recent foreign body ingestion?

Relieving factors

Is swallowing easier in a different posture?

Dysphagia

What do you think is wrong?

Ask about treatment already received.

Ask about CVAs in the past. (Cardiovascular risk factors)

➤ Past medical history

Have you had previous chest infections from aspiration?

Is there a history of indigestion, or peptic ulceration?

Have you had previous endoscopies?

Does the patient have any systemic conditions (eg scleroderma) or neurological disorders (eg myasthenia)?

Have you been treated before with dilatation therapy?

Is there a history of treatment with PPIs, H_2 antagonists?

Is there a history of operations for reflux (eg fundoplication)?

Is there a past history of polio/CVA?

Has there been exposure to radiation in that area (for breast cancer, Hodgkin's disease, etc)?

➤ Drug history

NSAIDs, alcohol – both may cause or exacerbate oesophagitis.

Have you taken *Helicobacter pylori* eradication treatment before?

➤ Social history

Do you smoke? How much? For how long? When did you stop?

Alcohol intake (GORD, gastritis, PUD).

➤ Family history

Is there a family history of oesophageal carcinoma or motor neurone disease?

➤ Differential diagnosis

Lesions of the mouth/pharynx

- Recurrent aphthous ulcers
- Stomatitis/glossitis/tonsillitis
- Quinsy/retropharyngeal abscess

Intraluminal

- Foreign body
- Polypoid tumours

Intramural

- **Peptic stricture (GORD)**
- **Carcinoma oesophagus/gastric cardia**
- **Infective (CMV, HSV, HIV, *Candida*)**
- Stricture secondary to ingestion of caustic substances or radiotherapy
- Pharyngeal/oesophageal web (Plummer–Vinson or George–Paterson–Brown–Kelly syndrome)
- Schatzki's (lower oesophageal) ring
- Pharyngeal pouch

Extrinsic compression

- Goitre with retrosternal extension
- Para-oesophageal (rolling) hiatus hernia
- Mediastinal tumours
- Enlarged lymph nodes
- Left atrial enlargement (mitral stenosis)
- 'Dysphagia lusoria' (compression from abnormally placed great vessels)

Motility disorders

- **Following CVA (stroke)**
- **Achalasia**
- **Diffuse oesophageal spasm**
- Scleroderma (part of the CREST syndrome)
- Parkinson's disease (hence sialorrhoea)
- Bulbar/pseudobulbar palsy
- Myasthenia gravis
- Motor neurone disease
- Hysteria (globus hystericus)

➤ Investigations

Blood tests

- Haematology – FBC, iron studies, ESR
    - Anaemia (malignancy, GI bleed (eg PUD), Plummer–Vinson)
    - Serum iron/TIBC/ferritin (Plummer–Vinson, GI bleed)
    - Raised WCC (infection)
    - ESR (malignancy, scleroderma)
- Biochemistry
    - U+Es (dehydration)
    - TFTs (goitre)
    - Glucose (modifiable risk factor if CVA)
    - CRP (infection)
    - LFTs (liver metastases)
    - Lipid profile (modifiable risk factor if CVA)
- Immunology
    - Autoantibody screen (scleroderma)

Microbiology

- Throat swab (pharyngeal lesions)
- Faecal occult blood (carcinoma, bleeding PUD)

Radiology

- CXR (AP and lateral)
  - Thyroid goitre extension
  - Left atrial enlargement
  - Tumours
  - Foreign body
  - Aspiration
  - Achalasia (air–fluid level behind heart)
  - Thoracic aortic aneurysm
- USS neck (thyroid goitre)
- Barium swallow (only if there is no absolute dysphagia for liquids; otherwise there is a risk of aspiration)
  - Motility disorder (eg achalasia)
  - Pharyngeal pouch (OGD risks perforation!)
  - Benign/malignant stricture
  - External compression
- CT thorax
  - Staging of tumour
- OGD ± biopsy and *Helicobacter pylori* status
  - Diagnostic
    - ➤ Malignant stricture (tumour)
    - ➤ Benign peptic stricture
    - ➤ Oesophagitis (inflammatory/infective)
    - ➤ Achalasia
    - ➤ Foreign body
  - Therapeutic
    - ➤ Balloon dilatation
  - Surveillance
    - ➤ Barrett's oesophagus (pre-malignant)

Further investigations

- Oesophageal endoluminal USS (staging oesophageal carcinoma)
- Bronchoscopy/mediastinoscopy (assessment of invasion of oesophageal carcinoma)
- Liver USS (staging of carcinoma)
- Laparoscopy (staging of carcinoma)
- Carotid Doppler (CVA)
- ECG (left atrial enlargement)
- Echocardiography (mitral stenosis, left atrial enlargement, CVA)
- CT brain (CVA)
- MRI brain (compression resulting in pseudobulbar palsy)
- Oesophageal manometry (oesophageal spasm)
- 24-hour oesophageal pH monitoring (oesophageal reflux)
- Anti-nAChR Antibodies (myasthenia gravis)
- Nerve conduction studies (motor neurone disease)
- Electromyography (motor neurone disease, myasthenia)
- Tensilon® test (myasthenia)

Dysuria

➤ History of presenting complaint

Onset

When is the pain or discomfort? Whilst or during attempting to urinate?

Duration – how long have you had it for?

Character

Distinguish actual burning pain in the urethra whilst passing urine (true dysuria), from exacerbation of abdominal pain whilst urinating as a result of movement of the bladder irritating the local peritoneum (peritonism).

Associated symptoms

Is there associated:

- haematuria
- penile or vaginal discharge
- cloudy urine
- offensive smelling urine
- urgency
- passage of grit or calculi
- loin pain
- abdominal pain
- suprapubic pain
- strangury (strong desire to urinate)

Urinary symptoms:

- hesitancy
- poor stream
- terminal dribbling
- incontinence
- increased/decreased frequency

Systemic features:

- weight loss
- fever
- sweats
- confusion
- malaise
- rigors (severe shaking)

Precipitating factors

Has there been any recent:

- instrumentation/**urinary catheters**
- sexual intercourse
- dehydration

Relieving factors

Antibiotics, analgesia

Has a urine sample been sent for urinalysis?

Is there any possibility you could be **pregnant**? When was your LMP?

What do you think is wrong?

Ask about treatment, if any, already received?

➤ Past medical history

Has there been any previous episodes of dysuria, UTIs, urinary calculi or renal disease? **Are you diabetic**?

Is there a history of gynae problems?

Has there been any recent instrumentation/indwelling catheters?

Did you have UTIs as a child, or have you had previous urinary tract **structural** problems?

Are you immunosuppressed? (increased risk UTI, renal TB etc)

Have you had **stones in the past**?

Have you had previous infective endocarditis? (UTI/renal abscess can be acquired via the haematogenous route)

➤ Drug history

Are you taking any antibiotic treatment?

Do you have any allergies to any antibiotics?

Is the elderly patient on HRT? (urogenital ageing, atrophic vaginitis)

➤ Social history

Do you use recreational drugs? (IE)

Sexual history? Have you had recent unprotected sex?

➤ Family history

Is there a FHx of recurrent UTIs, particulary those associated with reflux nephropathy?

➤ Differential diagnosis

Kidney
- Renal abscess
- Renal TB
- Acute pyelonephritis (rare)

Bladder
- **Pyogenic cystitis**
- Interstitial cystitis
- Bladder calculus
- Bladder tumour
- Colovesical fistula

Prostate
- Prostatitis

Dysuria

Urethra

- Urethritis
  - *Chlamydia*
  - Gonococcal
  - *Trichomonas*
  - *Candida*
  - *Herpes simplex*
- Female urethral syndrome

Vagina

- Vaginitis
  - Atrophic (postmenopausal)
  - *Candida*
  - *Trichomonas*
  - Bacterial vaginosis

➤ Investigations

Blood tests

- **Haematology: FBC**
  - raised WCC (infection)
- **Biochemistry:**
  - **U+Es** (renal function, obstructive uropathy)
  - **Glucose** (diabetes mellitus)
  - **CRP** (infection)
- **Microbiology:**
  - **Blood cultures** (urosepsis)
  - **Urinary M,C&S** (UTI)
  - **Three consecutive early morning MSUs** (renal TB)

Urine (MSU)

- UTI
- Glucose (DM)
- Blood (calculus)
- Exfoliative cytology (carcinoma)

Radiology

- **Renal USS:**
  - obstructive uropathy
  - hydronephrosis
  - Renal collection/pyelonephritis
  - structural abnormality

Further investigations

- **Vaginal/urethral swabs**
- **Cystoscopy**
- **Intravenous urography (IVU)** (structural abnormality)
- **CT urography (CTU)**
- **Micturating cystourethrogram** (vesico-ureteric reflux, bladder or urethral pathology)
- **DMSA (dimercaptosuccinic acid) scan** (assess renal function from recurrent sepsis)

Earache (otalgia)

➤ History of presenting complaint

Site

Is it one or both ears?

Onset

Duration? How long have you had this for?

Character

Is the pain worse when the ear is poked or moved around? (external ear pathology)

Radiation

Referred pain

Associated symptoms

- irritation
- discharge (profuse/scanty?, blood?, is it foul-smelling?)
- deafness
- tinnitus
- vertigo
- facial weakness
- swellings behind the ear (mastoiditis)

Are there any lesions around the ear, or inside the mouth (cephalic herpes zoster/herpes zoster oticus/Ramsay Hunt syndrome)?

Are there any systemic symptoms – fever, rigors, weight loss, malaise, anorexia, lethargy, palpitations?

Precipitating factors

Do you go swimming often?

Is there a history of trauma?

Is there a history of a FB being inserted into the ear?

Is there a history of poking the ear with a FB, eg matchstick/hairgrip/cotton-wool buds/paperclips to remove wax?

Is there a history of a common cold, tonsillitis, adenoiditis, infectious diseases (children)?

Is there a history of sinusitis, airflight, scuba diving, barotraumas (middle-ear)?

Could this be **referred** pain:
- History dental problems
- TMJ dysfunction
- History tonsillitis
- Pharyngitis
- Sinusitis
- Neck pain
- Hoarse voice (laryngeal pathology)
- Difficulty in swallowing (quinsy)

Do you have any difficulty swallowing or pain on swallowing (latter tonsillitis/pharyngitis/quinsy)?

Do you have throat/tongue pain (glossopharyngeal neuralgia, tumour posterior 1/3 tongue)

Relieving factors

Antibiotics, analgesia

Severity

Quantity of analgesia?

Amount of time spent off school?

What do you think is wrong?

Ask about treatment, if any, already received?

➤ Past medical history

Have you had a tonsillectomy/adenoidectomy?

Have you had previous episodes of tonsillitis?

Have you had grommets inserted?

➤ Drug history

Do you take any medications?

Have you taken analgesia?

Have you had any recent courses of antibiotics?

➤ Social history

Do you smoke? (OM, laryngeal carcinoma)

Do the parents of children smoke? (ie are the children exposed to passive smoking which increases the risk of OM?)

Overseas travel history, aeroplane travel, swimming.

How do the symptoms interfere with your life (school work, working)?

What is the extent of the patient's disability?

➤ Differential diagnosis

External ear

- **Otitis externa**
- **Malignant otitis externa (DM)**
- **Trauma**
  - Barotrauma
  - cotton buds
  - Subperichondral haematoma
- **Boil, furuncle**
- Foreign body (eg impacted wax)
- Malignancy
- Ear canal eczema/seborrhoeic dermatitis
- Chondrodermatitis helicis nodularis

Middle ear

- **Otitis media**
- **Mastoiditis**
- **Cholesteatoma**
- Herpes zoster oticus (Ramsay Hunt syndrome)

Referred pain

- **Mouth**
  - Caries
  - Dental abscess
  - Impacted molar
- **Tongue**
  - Tumour of posterior one third
- **Temporomandibular joint**
  - TMJ Dysfunction
- **Oropharynx and piriform fossa**
  - Tonsillitis
  - Pharyngitis
  - Quinsy
  - Foreign body
  - Postoperative
  - Malignancy
  - Glossopharyngeal neuralgia
- **Nose and sinuses**
  - Sinusitis
  - Carcinoma (NPC)
- **Larynx and hypopharynx**
  - Inflammation
  - Carcinoma
- **Parotid gland**
  - Carcinoma
  - Calculus
  - Sialadenitis
- **Oesophageal**
  - Oesophagitis
  - Carcinoma

Earache (otalgia)

- **Cervical spine**
  - Spondylosis
- **Trigeminal neuralgia**
- **Skin**
  - *Herpes zoster*

➤ Investigations

Blood tests

- **Haematology: FBC, ESR**
  - Anaemia (malignancy)
  - raised WCC (tonsillitis, otitis media, acute mastoiditis)
  - ESR (malignancy, infection)
- **Biochemistry**
  - **Glucose** (malignant otitis externa)
  - **CRP** (infection)

Microbiology

- **Ear swab** (otitis externa, otitis media with discharge, furuncle)
- **Throat swab** (tonsillitis)

Urine dipstick

- **Glucose** (malignant otitis externa)

Radiology

- **Skull X-ray** (mastoiditis)
- **X-ray TMJ/teeth**
- **CT/MRI** (inner ear/temporal bone pathology, malignancy, mastoiditis)

Further investigations

- **Paul–Bunnell (Monospot) test** (EBV)
- **Panendoscopy ± Biopsy** (malignancy, inflammation, foreign body)
- **Cervical spine X-ray** (cervical spondylosis)

Facial pain

Always clarify what the patient means by facial pain as it can be misinterpreted as headache and vice versa

➤ History of presenting complaint

Site

Where is the pain? (but note pain can be referred, eg. pain around the ear can be referred from the skin, teeth, tonsils, pharynx, larynx and neck).

Is there tenderness over the maxilla (sinusitis, dental abscess, carcinoma of sinus)?

Onset

Duration?

Character

What is the pain like?

Are there paroxysms of sharp, lancinating pains in the distribution of the trigeminal nerve?

Is there a dull, aching quality? (infections of teeth, mastoid, ear).

Radiation

eg Trigeminal neuralgia

Associated symptoms

Are there tears? (lacrimal duct obstruction, eg NPC)

Is there otorrhoea and hearing loss (otitis media/externa)?

Is there nasal obstruction, rhinorrhoea and unilateral epistaxis (NPC, maxillary sinusitis and carcinoma maxillary antrum)

Facial pain

Is there swelling of the cheek? (dental abscess, maxillary sinus carcinoma)

Is there proximal muscle weakness and pain (GCA with associated PMR)

Is there parasthesia in the distribution of the trigeminal nerve (often precedes vesicular rash of *Herpes zoster*)?

Is there any facial weakness? (*Herpes zoster*)

What about headaches?

Precipitating factors

What brings the pain on –

- **Food or chewing**? (dental abscess, salivary gland/duct disorder, TMJ disorder, GCA).
- Is the pain aggravated by **touch**? What about even the slightest touch/wind? (trigeminal neuralgia).

Are there any problems with teeth, sinuses or ears?

Relieving factors

Analgesia

What do you think is wrong?

Ask about treatment, if any, already received?

➤ Past medical history

Has there been any previous illnesses?

Have you had shingles/chickenpox in the past?

Do you suffer from depression/anxiety?

➤ Drug history

Do you take any medications?

> Social history

Occupation and lifestyle limitations due to condition.

> Differential diagnosis

Neurological

- **Trigeminal neuralgia**
  - Primary/idiopathic
  - Secondary/structural
    - > MS
    - > Arteriovenous malformation
    - > Acoustic neuroma
    - > Entrapment neuropathy (eg scleroderma)
- **Post-herpetic neuralgia**
- Glossopharyngeal neuralgia
- Cluster headache (migrainous neuralgia) and migraine
- Post-traumatic

Non-neurological

Cardiac

- **Cardiac pain (referred)**

Neck/pharynx

- Cervical disc pathology
- Tonsillar pathology
- Retropharyngeal mass (eg nasopharyngeal carcinoma)

Sinuses

- Sinusitis
- Neoplasia

Eye

- **Glaucoma**
- Iritis
- Optic neuritis
- Retro-orbital migraine
- Retro-orbital disease (eg cavernous sinus)
- **Posterior communicating artery aneurysm**
- Eye strain

TMJ

- Arthritis
- TMJ dysfunction and dislocation

Teeth

- Caries
- Dental abscess
- Malocclusion

Ear

- Otitis media
- Otitis externa
- Mastoiditis
- Parotid disease
    - Mumps
    - Parotitis
    - Duct obstruction (tumour/calculus)

Vascular

- **Giant cell arteritis**

Skin

- *Herpes zoster* (shingles)

Atypical facial pain

- A diagnosis of exclusion-linked with depression

> Investigations

Blood tests
- Haematology – FBC, ESR
  - Anaemia (malignancy)
  - Raised WCC (infection)
  - ESR (GCA, malignancy, infection)
- Biochemistry
  - U+Es (renal function)
  - CRP (infection)
  - Cardiac enzymes – Troponin I/T (MI)
- Virology
  - Herpes, mumps

Microbiology
- Ear swab/ mouth swab

ECG
- Angina, non-ST elevation MI, ST-elevation MI

Radiology
- Cervical spine X-ray
  - Cervical sponylosis
- Sinus X-ray
  - Sinusitis
  - Carcinoma sinus
  - Mastoiditis
- Dental plain film + TMJ Views
  - Dental carries, abscesses
  - TMJ
- USS ± FNAc (Parotid swelling)
- CT/MRI brain (MS/AVM/Posterior communicating artery aneurysm/ cerebellopontine angle tumour/carcinoma sinus/ nasopharyngeal carcinoma/parotid tumours)

Further investigations

- Lumbar puncture – Xanthochromia if aneurysm, oligoclonal bands (MS)
- Temporal artery biopsy (GCA)
- Sialography (parotid stones, sialectasis, tumour)
- Panendoscopy ± biopsy (pharyngeal tumour)

Faecal incontinence

➤ History of presenting complaint

Distinguish from **true diarrhoea** (see Chapter on Diarrhoea).

SOCRATES

Onset

Duration?

Onset (sudden/gradual?)

How often do you open your bowels?

Character

Do you have the feeling that your rectum is full?

Do you experience the urge to go?

Are you aware or unaware of soiling when it happens? (neuropathy)

Is there an overproduction of faeces and therefore is incontinence due to diarrhoea? (gastroenteritis is probably the commonest cause)

Associated symptoms

Is it associated with urinary incontinence (double incontinence)? (almost diagnostic of impaction as cause of both!)

Do you have any rectal bleeding?

Is there passage of mucus?

Have you had any changes in bowel habit?

Have you lost weight? How much? Over how long?

Do you have the sensation of something coming down? Is it when you pass stools? (piles, rectal prolapse)

Precipitating factors

Is there a history of trauma?

Is there a history of spinal cord injury?

Have you had any recent ano-rectal surgery?

Have you had any recent difficult childbirths – prolonged labour, forceps delivery, forceful delivery, perineal tears, episiotomy?

Is there a predisposition to peripheral neuropathy – DM, vitamin B_{12} deficiency, alcoholism, medications.

Is there a history of constipation (faecal impaction with overflow)?

Is there a history of recent stroke, dementia or neurological illness (eg MS)?

Relieving factors

Loperamide

Severity

Number of incontinence pads per day

How many times a day do you need to change your underwear because of soiling?

Do you soil the bed sheets at night?

What do you think is wrong?

Ask about treatment, if any, already received?

➤ Past medical history

Is there any history of previous illnesses?

Is there a history of IBD?

Is there a history of radiotherapy exposure?

➤ Drug history

Do you take any medications, such as laxatives or loperamide?

➤ Social history

Do you smoke?

Do you consume alcohol?

Do you use recreational drugs?

Overseas travel history, tropical illnesses.

Have you taken any time off work? How much?

How do the symptoms interfere with your life (walking, working, sleeping)?

➤ Family history

Is there a FHx of malignancy?

➤ Differential diagnosis

Gastrointestinal causes

All causes of diarrhoea (see Diarrhoea chapter) *plus*

- Overflow diarrhoea (faecal impaction, rectal neoplasm)
- Anal fistula
- Rectal prolapse
- Sphincter laxity
- Ano-rectal surgery (eg sphincterotomy, fistula-in-ano surgery)
- Third degree haemorrhoids
- Radiotherapy

Faecal incontinence

Non-gastrointestinal causes

Congenital

- Spina bifida
- Ano-rectal anomalies

Neurological

- Spinal cord compression
- Peripheral neuropathy (eg DM)
- Parkinson's disease
- Stroke
- Epilepsy
- Multiple sclerosis
- Trauma and tumours (brain, spinal cord, cauda equina)
- Dementia

Trauma

- Pelvic fractures
- Impalement

Obstetric

- Traumatic childbirth (puborectalis/nerve damage)

➤ Investigations

Blood tests

Haematology – FBC, haematinics, ESR

- Macrocytic anaemia (vitamin B_{12} deficiency → peripheral neuropathy)

Biochemistry

- Glucose (diabetes induced peripheral neuropathy)
- LFTs (alcohol induced peripheral neuropathy)

Urine dipstick

- Glucose (DM)

Proctoscopy

Sigmoidoscopy (biopsy)

Radiology

- MRI
  - Defects in ano-rectal mucosa
  - Pelvic malignancy
  - Spinal tumours
  - Spinal cord compression

Further investigations

- Endoanal USS (defect in ano-rectal mucosa)
- Ano-rectal manometry
- Electromyography (pudendal nerve neuropathy)
- Proctography
- EEG (epilepsy)

Falls and gait abnormalities

➤ History of presenting complaint

When and where did you collapse?

What were you doing at the time? (Standing, sitting, etc)

Did you lose consciousness, or not?

What was your premorbid/pre-fall health like?

Prior

How did you feel immediately prior to the episode?

Was there any warning or prodrome?

Did you trip over a loose carpet/rug/wires? Did you slip or were you pushed or pulled? Was the lighting poor? Was the floor slippery?

During

Did you sustain significant injury during the collapse? Did you injure your head during the fall?

What was the height from which you fell? (> Body height?)

Were you walking on the flat, going down stairs, turning, transferring or reaching when you fell?

Did you land on a hard surface? Did you fall sideways or straight down on your hip?

After

How did you feel afterwards?

Was there any weakness of any limb(s) afterwards?

Any previous episodes should be similarly analysed in detail.

Associated symptoms

Is there any pain now or before? Hip/legs, shoulder, head, dysuria, abdominal pain, pain on breathing, chest pain?

Do you have a headache?

Ask about:

- Aura
- Fits (Todd's paresis)
- Dizziness
- Vertigo
- Speech
- Hearing
- Sensation
- Numbness
- Tingling
- Diplopia

Are there any signs of raised ICP? (Space-occupying lesion, NPH)

Are the headaches worse with straining, sneezing or coughing? When are they worst? (In the morning?)

Are there associated changes in vision, nausea, vomiting, drowsiness?

Are there any disturbances of higher mental functioning, such as confusion? Is there any urinary/faecal incontinence? (NPH)

Associated systemic features:

- Fever
- Night sweats
- Rigors
- Weight loss
- Loss of appetite
- UTI (dysuria, frequency, urgency)

Precipitating factors

Vision – How is your eyesight/visual acuity? Do you have cataracts? Do you need new glasses? Do you have problems with your vision? (Amaurosis fugax/bits missing/flashing lights/floaters/painful eye/one eye or both eyes) When were your eyes last tested?

Gait – Do you have problems walking or inco-ordination? Do you have any pain/stiffness/deformity/swollen joints? (Arthritis) Limb weakness? Tremor? (At rest or when you do things?) Do you have postural instability?

Are there any features of cervical myelopathy? (Head movement restriction, arm pain, muscle wasting)

Ask about function:

- Do you have difficulty walking/doing things in the dark? (Proprioceptive loss)
- Do you find it difficult getting out chairs/reaching for items off the top shelf?
- Do you have difficulty walking/performing tasks?
- Have you been immobile for long periods of time/fractured a limb/been in a cast/not used a limb for a long time (eg arthritis)?

Cardiovascular risk factors

See Chest pain.

What do you think is wrong?

Ask about treatment, if any, already received.

➤ Past medical history

Is there any history of previous illnesses or operations, such as carotid endarterectomy?

What is your pre-morbid health like?

Previous neurological disorders?

Have you had previous falls, Parkinson's, dementia, MS, osteoporosis, carcinoma with bony secondaries (increased fracture risk from fall)?

Is there any history of cardiovascular conditions – MI/angina/chest pain, peripheral vascular disease/calf pain on walking, strokes/TIAs, renovascular disease?

Do you have arthritis/structural problems, including OA, RA, ankylosing spondylitis, cerebral palsy?

Do you have a previous history of trauma, fractures to lower limbs or polio, which could result in length inequalities? Is there a history of foot drop?

Do you have a bleeding disorder? (Would be a contraindication to taking aspirin or warfarin or could precipitate a subdural haemorrhage if he or she sustained a head injury)

➤ Drug history

Do you take any drugs that could cause or precipitate the event, or are you taking any drugs to treat a neurological disorder? (Phenytoin can precipitate cerebellar problems, for example)

➤ Social history

> Try to engage in the patient's pre-morbid functional status – be thorough!

What are the patient's disabilities?

What effect does the illness have on his or her life?

What would you like to do that you can't?

What has your condition prevented you from doing?

Who is at home with you and are they able to look after you?

Are you married/single? Do you have any children?

What help do you receive – relatives, neighbours, friends, social services, support workers, occupational therapists, district nurse?

What modifications, if any, have been made to your house?

Where do you live? (House, flat, bungalow, nursing home, residential home) What floor is your flat on? Is it warden-controlled? How many levels does your house have? Do you have stairs at home? What about stairs leading to the front door? Is there a lift in your block of flats? (Does it currently work?) Is your bedroom upstairs or downstairs?

Do you have to climb stairs to go to the toilet? Do you have any rails? Where? In the bedroom, bathroom, on the stairs? Can you bathe/shower/go to the toilet on your own? Can you get in and out easily? Can you dress yourself? Can you write independently?

Can you feed yourself and cook for yourself? What do you eat normally? Meals on wheels?

Do you have access to hot water, heating, electricity, a telephone?

Who does your washing?

Who does the housework?

How do you normally manage financially? Do you get a state pension? Do you get incapacity/unemployment/disability benefits?

Who does your shopping?

Do you get out of the house much? How do you normally spend your days? What are your hobbies (eg reading, watching TV)? Do you ever go to a day centre?

What was your mobility normally like prior to the fall? What about now? How far can you usually walk and what stops you? Do you walk unaided or with a walking aid? What do you use? (Stick, Zimmer frame, etc)

How do the symptoms interfere with your life?

➤ Family history

Is there a family history of neurological disease or arthritis?

➤ Differential diagnosis

Intrinsic causes

Medications/intoxications – most modifiable risk factor

- Antihypertensives and diuretics
- Benzodiazepines and other sedatives
- Antidepressants
- Levodopa
- Alcohol misuse

Cardiovascular

- Silent MI
- Arrhythmias
- Postural hypotension
- Syncope (carotid sinus, micturition, cough)
- Left ventricular outflow obstruction (aortic stenosis, HOCM)
- Dysbasia (eg intermittent claudication, ischaemia)

Sensory deficits

- Visual impairment (localised in eye or visual pathways)
- Vestibular problems (central or peripheral, Ménière's)
- Proprioceptive loss

Neurological

- Stroke
- Dementia/cognitive impairment
- Ataxia (cerebellar, proprioception)
- Epilepsy
- Cervical radiculomyelopathy
- Neuropathy (sensory, motor, autonomic)
- Drop attacks
- NPH

Gait disorders

- Parkinsonism
- Chorea

Musculoskeletal

- Deconditioning (weakness of legs/trunk secondary to disuse)
- Arthritis
- Previous fractures/osteoporosis/osteopenic vertebrae, myopathy
- Foot/shoe problems (eg bunion deformities)

Intercurrent acute illness

- Febrile illness (eg pneumonia, urosepsis)
- Hypothermia
- Dehydration

Falls and gait abnormalities

Extrinsic causes

Environmental hazards

- Slippery floor
- Poor lighting
- Household clutter (loose rugs, shiny/uneven/wet floor surfaces, lack of handrails, etc.)

Awkward movements

- Turning, transferring, reaching, stepping up/down

➤ Investigations

Blood tests

- Haematology – FBC, haematinics
  - Anaemia (exacerbates dizziness, postural hypotension)
  - Raised WCC (sepsis)
  - MCV (alcohol, hypothyroidism, vitamin B12 deficiency)
  - Haematinics (neuropathy)
- Biochemistry
  - U+Es (renal function, dehydration)
  - TFTs (hypothyroidism → cerebellar dysfunction)
  - Glucose (hypoglycaemia)
  - CRP (infection)
  - LFTs (alcohol)
  - Cardiac enzymes – troponin I/T (MI)
  - Digoxin levels and other drug assays

Microbiology

- Blood cultures (sepsis)
- Syphilis serology (VDRL)

Urine

- UTI
- Glucose (diabetes mellitus)

ECG

- Angina, MI
- Arrhythmia
- Conduction defect
- LVH (aortic stenosis, HOCM)
- 24-hour tape

Radiology

- CXR
  - Consolidation
- CT head
  - Ischaemia
  - Space-occupying lesion
  - Hydrocephalus
- MRI
  - Demyelination
  - Posterior fossa (cerebellar) pathology
- Echocardiography
  - Valvular dysfunction (especially aortic stenosis)
  - LV function
  - LVH

Further investigations

- Nerve conduction studies/EMG (peripheral neuropathy)
- Tilt table test (vasomotor syncope)
- Visual field analysis (perimetry) and slit lamp examination
- EEG (epilepsy)
- Lumbar puncture (NPH, MS)
- DEXA scan (osteoporosis increases fracture risk from falling)

Fatigue and lethargy

➤ History of presenting complaint

What do you mean by fatigue or tiredness?

Why have you sought medical attention now?

What do you think is wrong?

SOCRATES

Onset and duration

Character

Try to establish what they mean by tiredness – is it that they are unable to exercise, they have exertional breathlessness, or they are just fed up with life?

Is fatigue worse with activity and better with rest? (myasthenia gravis)

Associated symptoms

What were the first symptoms noticed?

What seemed to precipitate it?

Were there any significant social changes at this time?

Has there been any:

- Breathlessness
- Weight loss
- Fever
- Night sweats
- Loss appetite

Are there any features of anaemia:

- exertional breathlessness
- angina

Hypothyroidism:

- weight gain
- cold intolerance
- constipation
- menorrhagia

Diabetes mellitus:

- polyuria
- polydipsia
- weight loss
- infections

Addison's disease:

- dizziness
- poor appetite
- vomiting

Underlying malignancy:

- weight loss
- reduced appetite

Local symptoms:

- cough
- haemoptysis
- breast lump
- rectal bleeding
- change bowel habit

Renal failure:

- polyuria
- nocturia
- itch
- nausea
- vomiting

Cardiac failure:

- exertional SOB
- ankle oedema

Chronic infection:

- fever
- rigors
- night sweats
- poor appetite
- weight loss
- malaise

Polymyalgia rheumatica:

- Aches and pains
- Jaw claudication
- Visual changes
- Scalp tenderness
- Malaise
- Fever
- Weight loss

Osa/narcolepsy (morning headaches, daytime sleepiness, snoring)?

Are there any features of chronic fatigue syndrome:

- memory difficulties
- headaches
- myalgia
- sore throat with fatigue for over 6 months

Are there any features of psychiatric illness?

- depression
- anorexia
- lowered mood
- anhedonia
- early morning awakening
- suicidal ideation

Timing

Do you feel tired the whole time?

Precipitating factors

Alcohol, or substance abuse? (Are there/Have there been problems with alcohol dependence?)

Relieving factors

Relaxation, hobbies, exercise

Severity

Difficulty sleeping

What are you unable to do that you would like to do?

➤ Past medical history

Is there any history of serious illnesses in the past, psychological problems, psychiatric illnesses or previous episodes of fatigue?

➤ Drug history

Do you take any medications, such as beta-blockers?

A full family and social history is essential.

➤ Social history

Do you smoke? How much and for how long?

Do you consume much alcohol?

Do you use recreational drugs?

Life stressors – family, relationships, work, financial, moving house, health.

Overseas travel history, tropical illnesses.

Occupation (and its exposures), exercise capacity, lifestyle limitations due to disease.

How far can you usually walk, what stops you?

How do the symptoms interfere with your life (walking, working, sleeping)?

➤ Differential diagnosis

Physical

- Haematological: **anaemia**, blood dyscrasias
- Cardiac disease
- Respiratory: **obstructive sleep apnoea**, asthma (nocturnal symptoms)
- Oncological: **carcinoma**, lymphoma
- Gastroenterological: cirrhosis, hepatitis, IBD, peptic ulcer disase
- Endocrine: **hypothyroidism**, diabetes mellitus, hyperparathyroidism, hypopituitarism, Addison's disease
- Infectious: HIV, EBV, TB
- Electrolyte abnormalities: hypokalaemia, hyponatraemia
- Neurological: head injury, MS, myasthenia gravis, Parkinson's
- Rheumatological: RA, SLE, polymyalgia rheumatica

Physician Induced

- Post-operative
- Prolonged bed rest/physical deconditioning
- Radiotherapy
- Drug treatments (anticonvulsants, antidepressants, benzodiazepines, **beta-blockers**, chemotherapy, cytokines/interferons, hypnotics, neuroleptics, statins, steroids)

Physiological

- Pregnancy
- **Sleep disorders**: insomnia, shift work, jet lag, noise disrupting sleep
- Environmental: extreme temperature, high altitude, overexertion

Fatigue and lethargy

Psychiatric

- Alcohol and drug misuse/dependence
- Anxiety disorders
- Delirium/dementia
- Depression
- Eating disorders
- Schizophrenia
- Somatisation disorder

Psychosocial

- Bereavement, marital separation, worry disrupting sleep (work, relationships/family, financial, health, moving house)

Proposed (unknown aetiology)

- Chronic fatigue syndrome (ME), fibromyalgia, hyperventilation syndrome, IBS

➤ Investigations

Blood tests

- Haematology – FBC, ESR, blood film
  - Anaemia (microcytic, macrocytic or normocytic)
  - Raised WCC (infection, inflammation)
  - MCV (elevated in hypothyroidism and alcohol abuse)
  - ESR (infection, inflammation, malignancy)
  - Blood film (blood dyscrasia)
- Biochemistry:
  - U+Es (renal failure, Addison's, electrolyte anomalies)
  - TFTs (hypothyroidism)
  - (Addison's)
  - CRP (infection, inflammation)
  - CPK (hypothyroidism, inflammatory myopathies)
  - LFTs (liver failure, malignancy, alcohol, hepatitis)
  - Short synacthen test (Addison's)

ECG

- Ischaemia/infarct
- Arrhythmia

Urinalysis

- Glucose (DM)
- 24-hour urinary creatinine and protein (renal function)

Radiology

- CXR:
  - Cardiac failure
  - Malignancy
  - TB
- Echocardiography
  - LV function (CCF)

Further investigations

- Anti-nAChR antibodies (myasthenia gravis)
- Paul–Bunnell (Monospot) test (EBV)
- AAFBs, HIV testing
- Rheumatoid factor (arthritides)
- Autoantibody screen (connective tissue disease)
- Angiography (peripheral vascular disease)
- Electromyography and muscle biopsy (myopathies)
- Polysomnography/sleep studies (OSA)

Haematuria

➤ History of presenting complaint

Is the blood definitely in the urine and not coming from the vagina (menstruation) or rectum?

Is it true haematuria and not red urine from drugs (such as rifampicin), beetroot, or systemic diseases such as porphyria or rhabdomyolysis?

SOCRATES

Onset

How long have you had it?

Is it all the time, or only sometimes/intermittent?

What effect does exercise have on it?

Has haematuria been noticed previously? (With a dipstick during medicals?)

Character

Nature of bleeding?

Is it macroscopic or microscopic?

Is the urine smoky? (Suggests GN)

Is the urine brown? (If urine stands for while)

Are there any clots in the urine? (Elongated, ribbon clots suggest a pelvi-ureteric cause, ie from above the bladder, whereas clots that form in the bladder tend to be larger and more rounded in appearance)

Where in the stream is the blood noticed:

- Throughout (bladder, ureters, kidneys)
- Beginning (in otherwise clear stream – urethra, prostate)
- Just terminally (unusual – schistosomiasis, prostate, bladder base)

Haematuria

Associated symptoms

Does it occur after exercise? (Normal variant) How many times?

Does the urine contain crystals, stones or gravel? (Urinary stones)

Ask about any infective symptoms:

- Dysuria
- Fever
- Sweating
- Frequency

Is there loin pain? (Colicky or constant – stones vs pyelonephritis)

Or pain elsewhere? Has the pain moved with time?

Is there any strangury, ie do you have the desire to pass something that will not pass? (Stones)

Is the urine frothy? (Proteinuria)

Ask about any other symptoms, such as:

- Hesitancy
- Poor stream
- Terminal dribbling
- Nocturia
- Incontinence

Renal carcinoma

- Are there any abdominal masses?
- Are there any systemic features, such as weight loss, nausea and anorexia, vomiting?

Hypercalcaemic symptoms

- Vomiting
- Abdominal pain

Uraemic symptoms

- Nausea
- Itching
- Hiccups
- Lethargy
- Numbness (neuropathy)

Is there a history of trauma, say to the back?

Haematuria

Has there been a recent renal biopsy?

Is there a history of pharyngitis/myalgia before the problem started? (Suggests IgA nephropathy, post-streptococcal GN or HSP)

Is there arthralgia or are there skin rashes? (HSP)

Is there any bleeding anywhere else? Do you bruise easily? (Vasculitides)

Respiratory symptoms (Goodpasture's, PAN, Wegener's)
- Cough
- Sputum
- Fever
- Haemoptysis

Cardiovascular symptoms (infective endocarditis, AF leading to renal infarct)
- Palpitations
- Chest pain

GI symptoms (carcinoma prostate with local invasion into bowel, vasculitides)
- Change in bowel habit
- Rectal bleeding

Precipitating factors

Is there a history of traumatic episodes, eg urethral catheterisation?

Severity

Tiredness, dizziness on standing? (Suggesting anaemia)

What do you think is wrong?

Ask about treatment, if any, already received.

➤ Past medical history

Is there any history of previous similar episodes, prostatism or other diseases that affect the urinary tract?

Previous stones/UTIs?

Is there a past history of high blood calcium?

Is there a history of bleeding disorders, such as haemophilia?

Is there a history of sickle cell anaemia?

Have you previously been exposed to radiotherapy?

Is there a history of renal failure or hypertension?

Is there a history of infective endocarditis or acute intermittent porphyria?

➤ Drug history

Are you taking any medications?

Chronic/abusive use of analgesics? (Papillary necrosis)

Anticoagulants? (Although often coincidental pathology present!)

Are you taking any antihypertensives?

Compliance, side-effect(s) of medication, OTC/herbal remedies, allergies, eg contrast medium.

(What happens?)

➤ Social history

Do you smoke? (Risk factor for cancer) How much and for how long? When did you stop? (Ask if they have tried to stop, or congratulate them for stopping)

Do you consume much alcohol?

Do you use recreational drugs? (Vasculitides, infective endocarditis)

Have you come into contact with any person who has TB? (Renal TB)

Have you been abroad? (Overseas travel history, tropical illnesses)

- Have you been exposed to schistosomiasis?
- Have you been swimming in fresh water abroad?
- Have you been to any **malarial** zones in the last year?

Ask about occupation (occupational exposures), such as alanine dye industry, dry cleaners.

➤ Family history

Is there a family history of any renal diseases, such as polycystic kidney disease?

Do episodes of bloody urine run in the family? (Benign familial haematuria)

Is there a family history of deafness? (Alport's syndrome)

Is there a family history of sickle cell anaemia? (Or other haemolytic anaemias)

Is there any consanguinity? *Draw a family tree.*

➤ Differential diagnosis

General

- Menses in women
- Beetroot ingestion (beeturia)
- Strenuous exercise
- Bleeding diatheses, eg anticoagulants, haemophilia, thrombocytopenia
- Haemoglobinuria/myoglobinuria (haemolysis/rhabdomyolysis)
- Trauma (urethral catheterisation)
- Loin pain – haematuria syndrome

Local

Kidney

- **Blunt injury and trauma (including renal biopsy)**
- **Pyelonephritis**
- **Renal cell carcinoma**
- **Renal calculus**
- Renal infarction (eg embolus, infective endocarditis, renal vein thrombosis)
- Glomerulonephritis (commonly IgA nephropathy)
- Henoch–Schönlein purpura
- Renal TB
- Cystic renal disease
- Papillary necrosis

Ureter
- **Calculus**
- Tumour

Bladder
- **Trauma**
- **Cystitis**
- **Calculus**
- **Tumour (usually transitional cell)**
- *Schistosoma haematobium*
- Drugs (eg cyclophosphamide causes a haemorrhagic cystitis)

Prostate
- BPH
- **Carcinoma prostate**
- Prostatitis

Urethra
- Trauma
- Calculus
- Carcinoma
- Stricture
- Urethritis

➤ Investigations

Blood tests
- Haematology – FBC, clotting, ESR, blood film, cross-match/G+S
  - Anaemia (gross haematuria, malignancy)
  - Polycythaemia (RCC)
  - Raised WCC (infection)
  - Thrombocytopenia (blood dyscrasias)
  - Clotting (anticoagulants, blood dyscrasias)
  - ESR (malignancy, TB)
  - Blood film (haemolysis causing haemoglobinuria, malarial blackwater fever)
  - Cross-match/G+S (severe bleed)

- Biochemistry
  - U+Es (renal function)
  - Ca^{2+} (malignancy, calculi, reduced in rhabdomyolysis)
  - LFTs (malignancy)
  - CPK (rhabdomyolysis → myoglobinuria)
  - PSA (BPH, carcinoma prostate)

Microbiology

- Urethral swabs (urethritis)

Urinalysis

- Urine microscopy
  - Presence of intact red blood cells excludes haemoglobinuria, myoglobinuria and ingested substances
  - Red cell casts (glomerulonephritis)
- Pus cells and nitrite (infection)
- Pus cells alone (urethritis, TB, bladder tumour, interstitial cystitis)
- Protein alone (suggests renal disease)
- 24-hour urinary creatinine and protein (renal function)
- Exfoliative urinary cytology (carcinoma)
- Three consecutive early-morning MSUs (renal TB)
- *Schistosoma* eggs (schistosomiasis)

Radiology

- CXR
  - Cannonball metastases (RCC)
  - TB
- KUB (kidney, ureter, bladder – plain X-ray)
  - Renal calculus (90% radio-opaque)
- Renal USS
  - Carcinoma
  - Polycystic kidneys
  - Obstructive uropathy (calculus)
  - Trauma
- Intravenous urography (IVU) – now obsolete
- Transrectal USS ± prostatic biopsy (carcinoma prostate)

- CT
  - Staging for malignancy
  - CT urography (calculi)
  - Trauma

Further investigations

- Cystoscopy ± biopsy (carcinoma, infection, stone, interstitial cystitis)
  - Diagnostic
  - Therapeutic
  - Surveillance
- Ureteroscopy ± contrast visualisation (retrograde pyelography) (tumour, obstruction)
- Renal biopsy (glomerulonephritis, tumour)
- Selective renal angiography (renal AVM, tumour, trauma)
- Autoimmune screen (glomerulonephritis)
- Hb electrophoresis (sickle cell anaemia)
- DMSA scan (quantify each kidney's contribution to renal function as pre-operative measure)

Haemoptysis

➤ History of presenting complaint

First establish what the patient actually means by haemoptysis.

Are you sure you are not **vomiting** blood instead of coughing up blood?

Is the blood instead coming from the **upper nasal passages**? (Nose bleeds, bleeding in mouth, so called **pseudohaemoptysis**)

SOCRATES

Onset

When was this first noticed? (Sudden/gradual/chronic recurrent)

Duration?

Has it been one episode or several episodes?

Is it continuous/daily or intermittent?

Have you had it previously?

Character

How much blood have you expectorated? (Large volumes or traces of blood; eggcupful or spoonful; > 200 ml/24 h = high mortality)

What colour is it? (Pink sputum implies very small amounts of blood, fresh red, discoloured brown or rusty, mixed in with sputum/blood-streaked)

Is it fresh blood or specks of blood?

Is it definitely blood and not charcoal bits/coal? (Melanoptysis – seen in coal-worker's pneumoconiosis)

Associated symptoms

Is there associated cough, breathlessness, sputum production?

Is the sputum purulent? What is the smell/taste like? Is sputum long-standing?

Is breathlessness chronic or acute? (Latter PE, infection)

Is it worse on lying down? (Pulmonary oedema)

How many pillows do you sleep with? Has there been any PND?

Is there associated chest pain? (PE)

Is it worse on breathing? (Pleuritic) What about breathing deeply?

Do you have palpitations? (Mitral stenosis, PE)

Do you suffer from syncope? (PE)

Is there any leg swelling suggestive of a DVT?

Is there any weight loss or night sweats? (TB, carcinoma)

Is there any haematuria? Epistaxis? (HHT, Wegener's) Or bleeding elsewhere?

Precipitating factors

Are you a smoker? (Risk factor for carcinoma)

Risk factors for DVT/PE – especially recent surgery and/or prolonged immobility.

Have you had a recent throat or chest infection (URTI/LRTI)?

Have you been in contact with anyone with TB?

Is there any history of trauma to the chest or foreign body inhalation?

What do you think is wrong?

Ask about treatment, if any, already received.

➤ Past medical history

Is there any history of previous illnesses?

Is there a history of any coagulation disorders, such as haemophilia?

Have you had previous rheumatic fever? (Predisposes to mitral stenosis)

Have you had previous TB or TB treatment?

Is there a history of cardiac or pulmonary disease, childhood pneumonias, TB, bleeding disorders?

Is there coexisting renal disease? (Goodpasture's, Wegener's)

➤ Drug history

Are you taking any medications, such as anticoagulants?

Compliance, side-effect(s) of medication, OTC/herbal remedies, allergies. (What happens?)

➤ Social history

Do you smoke? How much and for how long? When did you stop? (Ask if they have tried to stop, or congratulate them for stopping)

Have you been abroad? (Overseas travel history, tropical illnesses)

Occupation? (Occupational exposures and asbestos exposure)

How far can you usually walk and what stops you?

How do the symptoms interfere with your life? (Working, sleeping)

➤ Family history

Is there a family history of malignancy?

Is there a family history of coagulopathies?

➤ Differential diagnosis

General

- Bleeding diatheses
- Exclude **spurious haemoptysis** (nose bleed, oral bleed, upper GI bleed)

Local causes

Cardiovascular

- **Pulmonary oedema**
- Mitral stenosis
- Aortic aneurysm
- Eisenmenger's syndrome

Respiratory

- Traumatic
    - Wounds
    - Post-intubation
    - Foreign body
- Infective
    - **Acute bronchitis**
    - **Pneumonia**
    - Lung abscess
    - **Bronchiectasis**
    - TB
    - Fungi
    - Paragonimiasis
- Neoplastic
    - **Primary**
    - Secondary
- Vascular
    - Infarction (thromboembolic disease)
    - Vasculitis
    - Wegener's
    - RA
    - SLE
    - PAN
    - Osler–Weber–Rendu disease
    - Arteriovenous malformation
    - Endometrioma (catamenial haemoptysis)

- Parenchymal
  - Diffuse interstitial fibrosis
  - Sarcoidosis
  - Haemosiderosis
  - Goodpasture's syndrome
  - Cystic fibrosis

> Investigations

Blood tests

- Haematology – FBC, clotting, D-dimers, ESR, cross-match/G+S
  - Anaemia (blood loss, malignancy, LVF)
  - Raised WCC (infection)
  - Clotting (exacerbates bleeding)
  - D-dimers (PE)
  - ESR (raised in carcinoma, sarcoidosis, infection, inflammation)
  - Cross-match/G+S (severe bleed)
- Biochemistry
- U+Es (pre-renal from blood loss, renal failure from vasculitis)
  - Ca^{2+} (raised in malignancy and sarcoid)
  - CRP (infection)
  - LFTs (metastases, cardiac cirrhosis)
  - Serum ACE (sarcoidosis)
- Immunology
  - Vasculitic screen (Wegener's, RA, SLE, PAN)
  - Anti-glomerular basement membrane antibodies (Goodpasture's)
  - Immunoglobulins (sarcoidosis)
- Arterial blood gases (PE, pneumonia)

Microbiology

- Blood cultures (pneumonia)
- Atypical serology (pneumonia)
- Heaf/Mantoux test (TB)
- Sputum M,C+S (infection, AAFBs, cytology)
- *Aspergillus* precipitins
- Three consecutive early-morning MSUs (TB)
- Gastric washings (TB)

Urinalysis

- Protein, red cell casts (glomerulonephritis – Wegener's, Goodpasture's)

ECG

- Sinus tachycardia (PE, blood loss)
- $S_1Q_3T_3$ (PE)

Radiology

- CXR
  - Consolidation
  - Bronchiectasis
  - TB
  - Pulmonary oedema
  - PE
  - Neoplasm (primary or secondaries)
  - Left atrial enlargement
- V/Q scan or CTPA (pulmonary embolus)
- (High-resolution) CT thorax ± percutaneous biopsy
  - Staging for neoplasia
  - Bronchiectasis
  - Interstitial lung disease
- Echocardiography
  - Mitral stenosis
  - Eisenmenger's syndrome
  - LV function (pulmonary oedema)
  - Right-sided heart failure (PE)

- Fibre-optic bronchoscopy (carcinoma, sarcoidosis, TB, vasculitides)
  - Diagnostic and therapeutic
  - Cytology – bronchial brushings, washings, BAL
  - Biopsy (histology)

Further investigations

- Renal biopsy (glomerulonephritis)
- Sweat test and faecal elastase (cystic fibrosis)
- Pulmonary function tests (bronchitis, bronchiectasis, sarcoidosis, carcinoma pre-operative assessment)
- Mediastinoscopy/thoracoscopy
- Bone scan/PET scan (carcinoma)

Haemoptysis

Headaches

➤ History of presenting complaint

Site

Where is the pain located?

Is it one-sided or bilateral?

Is it focal or generalised?

Is it a central, tight band?

Onset

When did the pain start?

What were you doing when the pain started?

How quickly did it come on? (Instantaneous, seconds to minutes, minutes to hours)

Is there a history of very sudden onset, suggesting SAH?

Character

What is the pain like/how would you describe it – throbbing/pulsating, stabbing, aching, pressure/tightness, prickly, shooting like electricity/lancinating?

Is a headache like this unusual for you?

Is the pain continuous? (Tension) Or intermittent? (Migraines)

How many different types of headache do you experience? (Separate histories are necessary for all)

Radiation

Does the pain radiate? (To the orbits, down to the face, temporal area – GCA, neck)

What about pain in the jaw, TMJ, or teeth, which can all be referred?

Associated symptoms

What else have you noticed?

Was there syncope at the onset or loss of consciousness/associated drowsiness?

Did any symptoms precede or follow the headache, such as visual disturbances? (How long does it take to develop and how long does it usually last; positive symptoms such as lines/dots, as well as negative ones like holes missing in the field)

Feelings of being detached, nausea/vomiting, anorexia, sweating/fever, photophobia (migraine, meningitis, glaucoma), phonophobia, osmophobia/ smells?

Does anything make the pain worse? (Head movement)

Ask about neck stiffness, neurological deficit, lacrimation, red/droopy eye, stuffy/runny nose, convulsions, speech changes, pins and needles, numbness, weakness of limb(s), ataxia, diplopia, recent viral infection (latter two suggestive of encephalitis), walking changes, incontinence, forgetfulness, drowsiness (NPH).

Is the aura in one eye, or both eyes? (By cover test – former is amaurosis fugax)

Is health normal between attacks?

Have you had any recent ear infections, or sinusitis? (Abscess, meningitis)

Are there any features to suggest a pituitary mass? (Changes in vision, infertility, menstrual irregularity, galactorrhoea, loss of libido, impotence, loss of well-being, etc)

Features of raised ICP:

- Is the pain exacerbated by coughing/straining/laughing/sneezing/ lying down?
- Does the headache wake you up early in morning?
- Is there any vomiting? If so, is it projectile?

Features of meningitis:

- Is there any neck stiffness, photophobia, fever, drowsiness, non-blanching rash, N+V, confusion?
- Have you been in contact with anyone with suspected meningitis?

Features suggestive of PMR/GCA:

- Do you get pain on eating?
- Do you get shoulder girdle pain?
- Do you have difficulty reaching up to shelves?
- Do you get pain combing your hair?
- Is your scalp tender?
- Do you have any visual symptoms, including blindness?

Focal neurology:

- Are there any accompanying neurological symptoms? (Seizures, confusion, etc)
- Is there any change in personality or deterioration in mental abilities? (Tumour, encephalitis)

Timing

How long have you had the headaches for?

How long does each one last?

Have you had it before?

When do they occur? (During the mornings – think about raised ICP, PMR; at night – think about clusters, acute angle-closure glaucoma, tension headaches and migraine; when stressed, at work – tension headaches; at weekends, on holidays – migraine)

How frequently do they occur? (Episodic/daily/unremitting)

How many pain (or pain-free) days to do you have on average a day/week/month?

Is there a diurnal variation, or does it occur at similar times each day? (Cluster headaches)

Exacerbating/precipitating factors

What brings it on/what made the pain worse? (Sun/bright lights, tension, anxiety, standing up for long periods, coughing/straining/bending over/exertion, hunger, particular foods – red wine, cheese, chocolate, Chinese food, ice-cream, sex, menses – catamenial migraine, stress, exercise, alcohol, OCP, weather conditions, sleep deprivation)

Are you intolerant to noise/light/smells?

Have you been exposed to any new drugs/toxins, or have you taken an overdose of anything?

Is there a history of head trauma?

Relieving factors

What takes the pain away? (Rest, darkened/quiet room, analgesia, massage, exercise, eating, stress)

What do you do during the headache? (Rest – migraine, or move around – clusters)

How much is activity limited or prevented? Does it stop you working?

Severity

Is it getting worse/better/staying the same?

Is this the worst pain you have ever had? Score out of 10 compared with childbirth.

Get an idea of severity by asking: Do you need to rest, sleep or keep away from work because of it? Does it disrupt sleep?

What do you think the headaches are due to?

Concerns/anxieties/fears about recurrent attacks and/or their cause (eg being due to a brain tumour).

➤ Past medical history

MITJTHREADS

Do you suffer from glaucoma?

Is this patient immunocompromised, or have they had a previous malignancy?

Have you had previous headaches, especially migraines?

Have you had previous neurological conditions? Have you had any recent lumbar punctures?

Do you suffer from hypertension?

Have you had shingles in the past?

➤ Drug history

Ask about medication already used and in what manner? (NSAIDs, triptans)

Do you abuse anti-inflammatories?

Have you had any recent antibiotics? (LP negative in meningitis)

Are you on the pill? (Migraine, benign intracranial hypertension, cerebral venous thrombosis)

Is there history of GTN, nifedipine, or substance withdrawal?

➤ Social history

Have you had any meningitis vaccinations?

Recent overseas travel history, tropical illnesses. (Meningitis, cerebral malaria)

Is there any chance that you could be pregnant? (Eclampsia)

Relation to mental state (eg depression, stress).

➤ Family history

Is there a family history of sudden deaths? (SAH) Or meningitis?

Is there a family history of similar headaches, especially migraines?

Is there a family history of cerebral haemorrhage?

Is there a family history of malignancy?

Is there a family history of glaucoma?

➤ Systemic enquiry

Especially cardiology and neurology.

➤ Differential diagnosis

Acute

- **Head injury**
- **Meningitis/encephalitis**
- **Haemorrhage** – subarachnoid, intracranial
- **Cerebral venous thrombosis**
- **Giant cell/temporal arteritis**
- **Carotid/vertebral artery dissection**
- **Acute angle-closure glaucoma**
- **Malignant hypertension**
- Sepsis/systemic infection
- Eclampsia
- Cerebral malaria (in tropics)

Chronic/recurrent

- Tension-type headache
- Migraine
- Cluster headache (migrainous neuralgia)
- **Raised** ICP
  - Tumour
  - Cerebral abscess
  - Haematoma
  - Hydrocephalus
  - Benign intracranial hypertension
- **Reduced** ICP
  - Post-lumbar puncture
- **Normal**-pressure hydrocephalus
  - Rarely gives rise to headaches and normally presents as a triad of dementia, gait apraxia and urinary incontinence
- Rebound headache on stopping analgesics
- **Giant cell/temporal arteritis**
- Referred pain from cervical spondylosis
- Sinusitis
- Referred pain from other facial structures (jaw, teeth, neck, eyes, ears, and cranial nerve neuralgias)
- Drugs (GTN, nifedipine, substance withdrawal)

> Investigations

Blood tests
- Haematology – FBC, clotting, ESR
    - Anaemia (anaemia of chronic disease)
    - Raised WCC (meningitis, abscess, sinusitis, systemic infection)
    - Clotting (intracranial haemorrhage)
    - ESR raised in infection, temporal arteritis
- Biochemistry
    - U+Es (hypertensive headaches with renal disease, pituitary tumours)
    - CRP (infection, GCA)
    - LFTs (Paget's disease)

Microbiology
- Blood cultures (meningitis, systemic infections)
- Throat swab, stool culture (encephalitis, meningitis)

Lumbar puncture for CSF (TB, bacterial and viral meningitis, encephalitis, subarachnoid)
- Opening pressure (raised ICP, benign intracranial hypertension, NPH)
- M,C+S
- Biochemistry (glucose, protein)
- Virology
- Ziehl–Neelsen stain
- Culture and Indian ink for *Cryptococcus*
- Cytology
- Xanthochromia (oxyhaemoglobin, bilirubin)

Urinalysis
- Proteinuria (eclampsia if pregnant)

Tonometry (glaucoma)

Radiology

- Skull and cervical spine X-rays
  - Head injury
  - Cervical spondylosis
  - Frontal view for sinusitis
  - Paget's disease
- CT/MRI head
  - Space-occupying lesion (abscess, tumour, haematoma)
  - Subarachnoid haemorrhage
  - To exclude raised ICP prior to LP
  - Pituitary tumour
- Angiography (MRI, CT or intra-arterial) (subarachnoid haemorrhage if fit for surgery, cerebral venous sinus thrombosis)

Further investigations

- Temporal artery biopsy (GCA)
- Blood films – thick and thin (cerebral malaria)
- EEG (encephalitis, space-occupying lesion/epileptogenic focus)
- Pituitary hormone assays (prolactin, TFTs, LH/FSH, testosterone, synacthen test, 24-hour urinary free cortisol, growth hormone, glucose tolerance test, water deprivation test)
- Lupus anticoagulant, anticardiolipin antibodies (antiphospholipid syndrome)

Hearing loss

➤ History of presenting complaint

DURATION? Has it been from birth?

Is it UNILATERAL or BILATERAL?

Onset (was it sudden or gradual)?

- Sudden = FB, trauma, vascular event, Ménière's
- Gradual = otosclerosis, old age (presbyacusis)

Is loss progressive, fluctuating or improving?

Is deafness continuous or intermittent? (Latter = Ménière's).

Is there a history of TRAUMA or head injury?

What PRECIPITATED it?

- Recent infection (mumps, herpes, meningitis)
- Drugs
- Trauma
- High level noise

Associated symptoms

Is there any pain? (Otitis externa, otitis media, zoster, trauma, barotrauma, perforated ear drum).

Is there any tinnitus/ringing in the ears?

Is there any vertigo?

Is there any aural or nasal discharge?

Is there any fever?

Are there any neck lumps?

Is there any facial weakness?

Are there any other cranial nerve or neurological deficits such as:

- weakness
- balance problems
- loss of sensation on face

- dysphagia
- eye movement problems
- diplopia
- incoordination/ataxia
- intention tremor
- headaches
- fits (acoustic neuromas, SOLs)

Do you suffer with ear wax?

- What is the hearing like in group conversation? (If better think of conductive hearing loss such as otosclerosis, if worse think of sensorineural loss)

What do you think is wrong?

Ask about treatment, if any, already received?

➤ Past medical history

Is there any history of previous illnesses including strokes?

Are there any problems with ears or hearing at/from birth?

Have you been exposed to teratogenic substances/viruses when younger, such as maternal rubella, toxoplasmosis, CMV?

When were your ears last syringed?

➤ Drug history

Medications, especially ototoxic drugs (**frusemide, gentamicin, aspirin**).

➤ Social history

Occupation (**occupational exposures** such as loud noise)

Lifestyle limitations due to disease.

How do the symptoms interfere with your life (working, communicating)? Do you wear any hearing aids?

Hearing loss

➤ Family history

Is there a FHx of deafness? (otosclerosis)

➤ Differential diagnosis

Conductive

Congenital

- Auditory meatus atresia

Acquired

- Impacted ear wax
- Foreign body
- Infection: Otitis externa, otitis media, cholesteatoma
- Eustachian obstruction ('Glue ear', tumours, eg nasopharyngeal carcinoma)
- Trauma: perforation of the tympanic membrane, barotrauma
- Otosclerosis
- Paget's disease

Sensorineural

Congenital

- Infections (rubella, toxoplasmosis, CMV)
- Perinatal hypoxia
- Eclampsia
- Genetic (eg Alport's syndrome)

Acquired

- Presbyacusis (age-related)
- Trauma: noice induced, head injury, surgery
- Ototoxic drugs: aminoglycosides, aspirin, frusemide, cytotoxics
- Infections: meningitis, mumps, measles, influenza, *Herpes zoster*, syphilis (rare)
- **Tumours: Acoustic neuroma (vestibular schwannoma)**
- Labyrinthitis
- Ménière's disease
- Paget's disease

> Investigations

Microbiology

- Swab of ear discharge (refractory otitis externa)
- Rubella/CMV/toxoplasma serology

Age appropriate hearing test/audiometry

Impedance tympanometry

Radiology

- **MRI**
  - Acoustic neuroma
  - Brain tumour
  - MS

Further investigations

- **Skull X-ray** (Paget's disease)
- **Alkaline phosphatase** (Paget's disease)
- **FBC/haematinics** (Vitamin B12 deficiency)
- **Flexible nasopharyngoscopy ± biopsy, + skull base radiology** (nasopharyngeal carcinoma)

Hoarseness and voice disorders

➤ History of presenting complaint

Onset and duration

Have you had it before?

How did it start?

Is it getting worse/better/staying the same?

Character

What is the pattern – transient (infection, excessive vocal use, smoking, alcohol, chemical fumes), progressive (tumours), or sustained (recurrent laryngeal nerve palsy)?

Associated symptoms

Have you had a recent viral illness/flu?

Do you have a sore throat?

Do you have a cough? (when is it worse?)

Do you have a fever?

Do you have postnasal drip?

Do you have a neck swelling? (goitre)

Is there any dysphagia (oesophageal carcinoma, laryngeal carcinoma)?

Is your breathing noisy (stridor)? (goitre, lung carcinoma, laryngeal carcinoma)?

Do you aspirate or suffer from repeated chest infections?

Do you have referred ear pain? (laryngeal carcinoma)

Has there been any breathlessness, drooping of your eyelid or wasting of the small muscles of your hand (lung carcinoma)?

Is there any double vision or muscle fatigue/lethargy? (myasthenia gravis)

Are there any symptoms of GORD (regurgitation, waterbrash, acidbrash, heartburn, abdominal pain)?

Are there any symptoms of hypothyroidism/ myxoedema (weight gain, cold intolerance, constipation, menorrhagia)?

Are there any associated systemic features – fever, malaise, weight loss, jaundice?

Precipitating factors

Have you been overusing your voice recently, eg excessive singing/ shouting?

Is there a history of recent inhalational injury, eg exposure to smoke/fire?

Is there a history of blunt trauma to the larynx/ laryngeal fractures?

Has there been recent laryngeal intubation?

Ask abour risk factors for head and neck malignancy (squamous cell carcinoma):

> ➤ *Risk factors for head and neck malignancy*
>
> **S**moking (and betel nut chewing)
> **S**pirits (alcohol)
> **S**pices
> **S**ore/**S**harp tooth (dental caries)
> **S**yphilis
> **S**epsis

What do you think is wrong?

Ask about treatment, if any, already received?

➤ Past medical history

Have you had any previous illnesses or operations, especially thyroidectomy, parathyroid surgery, carotid endarterectomy, thoracic surgery?

Is there any history of thyroid disease or goitres?

Is there any history of malignancy, especially lung, oesophagus, larynx?

Is there a history of syphilis or Marfan's syndrome? (thoracic aortic aneurysm).

➤ Drug history

Do you take any medications?

Do you take ACE inhibitors (excessive coughing, triggers angioneurotic edema)?

Do you use steroid inhalers for asthma? Does it cause oral Candida, or thrush? Do you use a spacer device? Do you gargle after using your inhalers? How often do you use your inhalers?

Compliance, side-effect(s) of medication, OTC/herbal remedies, allergies. (What happens?)

➤ Social history

Do you smoke? How much and for how long? When did you stop? (Have you tried to stop, or congratulate them for stopping). Do you or have you ever chewed tobacco or betel nut? (risk factor for head and neck carcinoma)

Do you consume much alcohol?

Do you use recreational drugs?

Overseas travel history, tropical illnesses.

Occupation (occupational exposures), exercise capacity, lifestyle limitations due to disease.

Do you need a loud voice at work, do you make announcements?

Have you taken time off work? How much?

How far can you usually walk, what stops you?

How do the symptoms interfere with your life (walking, working, sleeping)?

➤ Family history

Is there a FHx of malignancy?

Has there been contact with TB or other infections?

➤ Differential diagnosis

Congenital

- Laryngeal web

Inflammation

- **Upper respiratory tract infection (laryngitis)**
- **Vocal cord strain**
- **Gastro-oesophageal reflux**
- **Postnasal drip**
- Allergies (angioedema)
- Chemical fumes

Neoplasia

- Benign:
  - **Singer's nodules**
  - **Papillomas/polyps**
  - **Goitre**
  - Acoustic neuroma
- **Malignant:**
  - **Larynx**
  - **Lung**
  - **Thyroid**
  - **Oesophagus**

Vascular

- Thoracic aortic aneurysm
- Superior vena cava syndrome
- Left atrial enlargement (Ortner's syndrome)
- Pulmonary oedema

Hoarseness and voice disorders

Intoxication

- **Smoking (Reinke's oedema)**
- Alcohol
- **Inhaled steroids** (asthma, COPD)
- **Unhumidified oxygen therapy**

Trauma

- Post-intubation
- Surgery
    - Thyroid
    - Parathyroid
    - Carotid endarterectomy
    - Thoracic

Endocrine

- **Myxoedema**
- Riedel's struma
- Hypoparathyroidism

Degenerative

- Myasthenia gravis
- Motor neurone disease

Psychogenic

- Hysterical dysphonia

➤ Investigations

Blood tests

- Haematology – FBC, ESR
    - Anaemia (malignancy)
    - White cell count (laryngitis)
    - ESR (laryngitis, malignancy)
- Biochemistry
    - TFTs (hypothyroidism)

Microbiology

- Throat swab

Radiology

- CXR and X-ray thoracic inlet:
  - Neoplasia
  - Thoracic lesions compressing recurrent laryngeal nerve
  - Widened mediastinum with thoracic aneurysm
- CT Neck:
  - Staging for laryngeal and thyroid carcinoma
- CT Thorax:
  - Lung tumours, thoracic aneurysms

Further investigations

- Direct/Indirect laryngoscopy
- 24-hour pH studies (oesophageal reflux)
- OGD (oesophagitis, oesophageal carcinoma)
- Tensilon® test (myasthenia gravis)
- Aortography (thoracic aneurysm)
- FNAc (thyroid carcinoma)
- Complement, C1 esterase inhibitor (angioneurotic oedema)

Hoarseness and voice disorders

Jaundice

➤ History of presenting complaint

First establish what the patient means by jaundice (some people think it means off-colour, ill or depressed).

SOCRATES

Onset

When was the jaundice first noticed?

How/why? By whom?

Character

Where is it? (Eyes, skin or both – only the eyes are affected in the early stages)

Is it continuous or intermittent? (An example of the latter is Gilbert's syndrome)

Is it getting better/worse/staying the same? (That is, is it **progressive**?)

Associated symptoms

Do you have any abdominal pain, fever, rigors, arthralgia, loss of appetite, weight loss (Do your clothes/belt feel looser?), swollen glands, anorexia, nausea, vomiting, steatorrhoea/altered bowel habit, dark urine/pale stools, pruritus, bruising, bronzed skin, rashes, upper/lower GI bleeding?

Malignant process

- *Are there any features suggesting malignancy?* (Change in bowel habit, weight loss, back pain, leg swelling)

Inflammatory bowel disease (PSC)

- Have you had any bowel symptoms, back pain, painful eyes or skin changes?

Chronic liver disease

- *Is there any abdominal swelling due to ascites, easy bruising, itchy skin, red pigmentation (spider naevi) or striae?*

Precipitating factors

Are there any precipitants? (Fasting and Gilbert's syndrome) Such as:

- Travel (malaria, hepatitis)
- Food (Have you eaten any seafood/dodgy food lately?)
- Contacts (Have you been in contact with anyone with jaundice?)
- Infective process (Have you had any recent infections? Have you had a sore throat, swollen glands, rashes, fever, arthralgia, abdominal tenderness?)

Other

Have you gone off your cigarettes? (Viral hepatitis)

Did you feel unwell at all prior to becoming yellow? (Hepatitis)

➤ Past medical history

MITJTHREADS

Have you been jaundiced before? *Is there a history of or known viral hepatitis/pancreatitis?*

Is there a history of chronic liver disease or malignancy? Have you had a GI bleed in the past?

Have you had any blood transfusions? Have you had any needle-stick injuries? *Homosexuality?* Have you come into contact with anyone with hepatitis?

Is there a recent history of surgery, *or exposure to halothane-based anaesthetics?*

Is there a history of known gallstones/*USS with gallstones, or previous cholecystectomy/biliary tract surgery?*

➤ Drug history

What medications do you take?

Have there been any **changes of medication recently**?

Consider all prescribed, illicit and alternative medications (can cause haemolysis, cholestasis and hepatitis/cirrhosis), especially paracetamol, the OCP and antibiotics such as co-amoxiclav.

Have you **overdosed** on any medications, eg paracetamol, as a suicide attempt or accidentally in an attempt to reduce arthritic pain?

➤ Social history

How much alcohol do you consume? Are you dependent on it?

CAGE questionnaire (see page 7).

Do you use, or have you ever used recreational drugs? Do you have any tattoos?

Have you ever been a recipient of blood products? In which country?

Have you been abroad? (Overseas travel history, tropical illnesses – yellow fever, malaria, etc). Were you ill while away? Did you eat shellfish? (Hepatitis A)

Have you been swimming in rat-infested waters? Have you been exposed to sewage, drains, outdoor water?

Occupation (occupational exposures – needle-stick injuries). Have you taken time off work? How much?

What are your hobbies? (Water sports?)

Sexual history (HIV, hepatitis) – First say, 'I need to ask you some important but rather personal questions.'

Have you been vaccinated against hepatitis A/B?

➤ Family history

Is there a family history of jaundice? (Haemolytic anaemias, haemochromatosis, Gilbert's syndrome, Crigler–Najjar) Liver problems? (Wilson's, α_1-antitrypsin deficiency) Diabetes mellitus? (Consider haemochromatosis)

Is there a family history of inflammatory bowel disease? (PSC)

Is there a family history of emphysema/lung disease? (α_1-antitrypsin deficiency)

Is there any consanguinity? *Draw a family tree.*

➤ Differential diagnosis

Pre-hepatic jaundice

- Haemolysis
- Gilbert's syndrome and other congenital enzymatic defects in bilirubin metabolism (eg Crigler–Najjar syndrome)
- Dyserythropoiesis

Hepatocellular jaundice (cirrhosis)

- Congenital/genetic – haemochromatosis, Wilson's, α_1-antitrypsin deficiency
- **Alcohol**
- Drugs and toxins
- Autoimmune, eg PBC
- **Infectious hepatitis** – viral hepatitis, leptospirosis, CMV, HIV, EBV
- **Carcinoma** – primary (hepatocellular carcinoma) and secondary/metastatic
- Cardiac cirrhosis – CCF

Post-hepatic jaundice

- **Gallstones** within the common bile duct
- **Carcinoma of the head of pancreas**
- **Ascending cholangitis**
- Carcinoma around the ampulla of Vater
- Lymphadenopathy at the porta hepatis
- Primary sclerosing cholangitis
- Mirizzi's syndrome
- Benign strictures of the common bile duct
  - Inflammatory (pancreatitis)
  - Post-operative
  - Post-radiotherapy
- Malignant strictures of the common bile duct (cholangiocarcinoma)
- Haemobilia

➤ Investigations

Blood tests

- Haematology – FBC, clotting, ESR, haematinics, blood film
  - Anaemia (haemolysis, malignancy)
  - MCV ↑ (alcohol, haemolysis)
  - Elevated WCC (hepatitis, ascending cholangitis)
  - Clotting (liver disease – prothrombin time prolonged in liver disease)
  - Serum iron and ferritin ↑ and TIBC ↓ (haemochromatosis)
  - Blood film (↑ reticulocytes in haemolysis)
  - ESR (infection, malignancy)
- Biochemistry
  - U+Es (hepatorenal syndrome)
  - LFTs – ALT, AST, ALP, bilirubin, GGT
  - Fractionated bilirubin (unconjugated and conjugated) (Gilbert's, Crigler–Najjar)
  - Glucose (chronic liver disease, diabetes in haemochromatosis)
  - Albumin (chronic liver disease)
  - CRP (infection, inflammation)

- Cholesterol (PBC)
- Amylase (pancreatitis → inflammatory CBD stricture, gallstone pancreatitis)
- Serum copper and caeruloplasmin (Wilson's disease)
- Paracetamol levels
- Immunology
  - Antimitochondrial antibodies (PBC)
  - Autoantibodies
    - IgM (PBC)
    - IgG (autoimmune hepatitis)
    - IgA (alcoholic liver disease)
    - ANA, anti-smooth muscle antibodies, LKM1 (autoimmune hepatitis)
  - Tumour markers
    - CA 19-9 (pancreas), CA 125
    - Serum α-fetoprotein (hepatocellular carcinoma)
    - CEA (bowel cancer with metastases)

Microbiology

- Hepatitis A/B/C, CMV, HIV, EBV serology
- Blood cultures (sepsis, leptospirosis)
- Leptospirosis complement fixation test

Urinalysis

- Urobilinogen (absent in obstructive jaundice)
- Conjugated bilirubin (absent in pre-hepatic causes)
- Haemoglobinuria, haemosiderinuria (haemolysis)
- M,C+S (leptospirosis)

Lumbar puncture (leptospirosis)

Radiology

- CXR
  - Enlarged heart (cardiac cirrhosis)
- AXR
  - Gallstones (though only 10% are radio-opaque)
  - Enlarged liver/spleen

- Transabdominal USS ± FNAC (liver, gallbladder, pancreas)
  - Gallstones
  - Dilated bile ducts
  - Pancreatic carcinoma
  - Hepatic masses/cirrhosis
  - Evidence of portal hypertension
- CT abdomen ± percutaneous biopsy
  - Pancreatitis
  - Staging for pancreatic carcinoma
  - Cholangiocarcinoma
- ERCP
  - Diagnostic (+ biopsy/brush cytology) – PSC, carcinoma head of pancreas, chronic pancreatitis, cholangiocarcinoma
  - Therapeutic – gallstone removal, palliative stent insertion in carcinoma head of pancreas
- PTC (if ERCP fails)
- MRCP (gallstones, pancreatic carcinoma, cholangiocarcinoma)
- Echocardiography (CCF)

Further investigations

- Serum haptoglobins, LDH, direct Coombs' test, chromium-labelled red blood cells (haemolysis)
- Serum α_1-antitrypsin levels
- Liver biopsy (hepatocellular disease, carcinoma)

Joint disorders (mono/polyarthritis)

➤ History of presenting complaint

Site

Is it symmetrical or asymmetrical?

Onset

Is it rapid or slowly progressive?

Has it changed with time? (Flitting arthritis)

How did the symptoms begin?

How long have you had the problem?

Character

What is the **main** joint problem?

- Pain
- Stiffness
- Swelling
- Deformity
- Loss of function
- Reduced mobility/limping

What bothers you **most**?

What joint or which joints are affected (wrists, fingers, elbows, shoulders, knees, ankles, atlanto-axial joint, back)?

Is it one or more joints?

Is it persistent or relapsing?

Radiation

Does the pain radiate elsewhere?

Associated symptoms

Do you have any **pain**? Where is the pain?

Are there any skin nodes or nodules?

Is there weakness? (With or without wasting of muscles)

Has there been any locking of the joint or instability (giving way)?

Have you had any recent infections? Are there any bowel symptoms (diarrhoea, abdominal pain, vomiting) or STIs (dysuria, genital discharge)?

Is there anyone with diarrhoea in the family? (Reiter's) What about previous sore throats? (Rheumatic fever)

Is there any eye pain/red eye, back pain? (AS)

Are there any skin changes/psoriasis/SLE?

Are there any features of IBD (Crohn's disease/UC) – diarrhoea, rectal bleeding, abdominal pain, vomiting, weight loss, fever, etc?

Are there any features of SLE – mouth ulcers, chest pain, fits, depression, history of thromboembolic events, Raynaud's (cold hands)? (Do your hands change colour at all?)

Are there any systemic features, eg skin rashes, ulcers, fever, rigors (septic arthritis), malaise, symptoms of anaemia, weight loss, dry eyes/mouth, breathlessness, numbness, paraesthesia (carpal tunnel), ankle swelling (nephrotic syndrome secondary to RA treatment)?

Timing

When do you get the pain and/or stiffness? (During cold weather, at the end of the day, in the morning upon wakening, after prolonged rest, during/after exercise, at night?)

How long does the morning stiffness last? (Just a few minutes indicates 'joint gelling' associated with degenerative disease; longer than 15–30 minutes of morning stiffness indicates inflammatory conditions such as RA, AS, PMR)

Precipitating/relieving factors

Was there trauma to the joint?

Did it coincide with starting any medications? (SLE)

When are the symptoms worse? When in the day are the symptoms worst?

What exacerbates them?

Does exercise make it better (inflammatory cause) or worse (mechanical)?

Is there a history of an infected lesion, such as ingrowing toenail/boil/ulcerating lesion?

Severity

What are the functional consequences, eg unable to walk, rise from a chair or write a letter?

What do you think is wrong?

Ask about treatment, if any, already received.

Past medical history

Is there any history of previous joint problems – rheumatism, arthritis or gout?

What has been the pattern of disease?

What was the age of onset?

What joints have been affected?

What is the activity like?

How long do episodes usually last?

Are any other organs involved, such as the heart (aortic stenosis)?

Have you had any joints replaced? Do you see a physiotherapist? Do you use any aids? Have you had any response?

Have you had any recent fractures?

Do you suffer from osteoporosis?

Joint disorders (mono/polyarthritis)

Is there any history of other serious illnesses or autoimmune disorders such as SLE, IBD or psoriasis?

Is there a history of renal failure (gout, SLE, RA drugs may cause renal failure), blood disorders, or psoriasis which can precipitate arthritis?

➤ Drug history

Have any medications been used to treat the joint(s)? (NSAIDs, antibiotics, allopurinol, corticosteroids)

Is there a history of corticosteroid or other immunosuppressant therapy?

Are you on any anticoagulant medications?

Does the patient use any drugs that may precipitate gout? (Such as thiazides, ciclosporin)

Compliance, side-effect(s) of medication, OTC/herbal remedies, allergies. (What happens?)

➤ Social history

Do you smoke? (Risk factor for OA) How much?

Do you consume alcohol? (Gout)

Do you use/have you used recreational drugs? (Viral hepatitis, septic arthritis, HIV)

Overseas travel history. Do you remember being bitten by an insect? (Lyme disease)

Occupation (occupational exposures), exercise capacity, lifestyle limitations due to disease?

Have you taken time off work? How much?

Are there any features of depression/feelings of helplessness?

How far can you usually walk and what stops you? What aids are you using? (Wheelchair, chair lift, home modifications)

How do the symptoms interfere with your life? (Walking, working, sleeping, feeding)

What are the social consequences of the joint problem? Can you walk or transfer independently? Can you dress, do up buttons, use cutlery or write independently? Has the disease affected work, family, spouse or children?

How has the joint disease affected you socially and at work, eg typing?

Have you tried any adaptations to try to improve mobility?

Sexual history – unprotected intercourse/risky sexual practices? (Reactive arthritis, viral hepatitis, HIV arthropathy)

➤ Family history

Is there a family history of musculoskeletal problems or arthritis?

Is there a family history of gout, psoriasis, AS, IBD?

Is there a family history of any other autoimmune disorders?

➤ Differential diagnosis

Monoarticular

- Septic arthritis
  - **Staphylococcal**
  - **Gonococcal**
  - **Gram-negative bacilli**
  - **TB**
  - **Lyme disease**
- **Gout**
- **Pseudogout (chondrocalcinosis)**
- **Traumatic haemarthrosis (haemophilia, trauma, loose body)**
- Palindromic RA
- Monoarthritic OA
- Seronegative arthritides (see polyarticular arthralgia)
- Malignancy (pigmented villonodular synovitis)
- Osteochondritis dissecans (loose body)

Polyarticular

- **Osteoarthritis**
- **RA**
- **Seronegative arthritides**
  - **Ankylosing spondylitis**
  - **Psoriatic**
  - **Reiter's/reactive**
  - **Enteropathic (IBD, Whipple's)**
  - **Behçet's**
- **Chronic polyarticular gout/pseudogout**
- Infections
  - **Bacterial** – gonococcal, meningococcal, endocarditis, TB, *Mycoplasma* pneumonia, Lyme, brucellosis
  - **Viral** – rubella, EBV, parvovirus B19, infectious hepatitis, HIV
- **PMR**
- Drug-associated (eg penicillins)
- Relapsing polychondritis
- Malignancy (hypertrophic pulmonary osteoarthropathy, leukaemia)
- Systemic diseases
  - **SLE**
  - Sarcoidosis
  - Sjögren's
  - Sickle cell disease
  - Rheumatic fever
  - HSP and other primary vasculitides
  - Haemochromatosis
  - Familial Mediterranean fever

Joint disorders (mono/polyarthritis)

> Investigations

Blood tests
- Haematology – FBC, clotting, ESR, haematinics
  - Anaemia (anaemia of chronic disease)
  - Raised WCC (septic arthritis)
  - Clotting (haemarthrosis – anticoagulant therapy, haemophilia)
  - ESR (chronic inflammation, infection)
  - Iron studies and ferritin (haemochromatosis)
- Biochemistry
  - U+Es (sepsis, renal failure via renal involvement in multisystem
  - connective tissue disease, eg SLE, urate nephropathy)
  - Ca^{2+} (chondrocalcinosis)
  - LFTs (hepatic involvement, eg haemochromatosis, viral hepatitis)
  - Glucose (diabetes mellitus and increased infection risk)
  - Serum urate (gout)
  - CRP (infection, elevated ESR and normal CRP = SLE)
  - PSA (carcinoma prostate)
  - CPK (inflammatory myopathies)
- Immunology
  - Rheumatoid factor
  - ANA (SLE)
  - ENA, eg anti-dsDNA (SLE)
  - Complement levels
  - HLA-B27 status

Microbiology
- Blood cultures (septic arthritis)
- Lyme/*Brucella* serology
- Viral serology – hepatitis/EBV/HIV/rubella
- Antistreptolysin O titre (rheumatic fever)

Joint aspirate

- Pus (septic arthritis)
- Blood (haemarthrosis)
- M,C+S
- Crystals (gout/pseudogout)

Urinalysis

- Proteinuria/haematuria (renal involvement in connective tissue disease, eg HSP)

Urethral/high-vaginal/throat/rectal swabs (gonorrhoea, Reiter's syndrome/reactive arthritis)

Radiology

- Local joint X-ray
  - Fracture
  - OA/RA/psoriatic/gout/ankylosing spondylitis
  - Avascular necrosis
  - Malignancy
  - Chondrocalcinosis
- USS joint
  - Effusion

Further investigations

- Arthroscopy
- Synovial biopsy (confirms types of arthritis in rare cases)
- Blood film/Hb electrophoresis (sickle cell anaemia)
- Serum ACE levels/Kveim test (sarcoidosis)
- CXR (bronchial carcinoma relating to hypertrophic pulmonary osteoarthropathy, TB)

Leg pain

Most of the following questions have been designed to tease apart the various neurological causes (especially spinal stenosis) from the vascular causes (such as intermittent claudication) – otherwise the two can be difficult to differentiate.

➤ History of presenting complaint

Site

Where is the pain?

Is it unilateral or bilateral? If both legs, which leg is worse?

Is the pain deep in the muscle or in the skin?

Is it the joints that hurt?

Onset

How long has the pain been present?

Did it come on? Suddenly? (DVT, acute ischaemia – embolus, trauma, etc) Or gradually?

Character

Is it getting better or worse?

When do you get the pain? (At night, at rest, during exercise, while putting shoes and socks on?)

What is the pain like?

Do you get shooting pains down the leg?

Radiation

Does it go anywhere else? Do you get any pain in the feet, calf, buttocks, back of the thighs?

Do you have any **back pain**?

Associated symptoms

Is the leg warm, tender, swollen? (DVT, cellulitis)

Is it cold, pale, numb? Pins and needles with loss of function, or mottling of the skin?

What is the pattern of numbness? (Dermatomal or stocking loss)

Are there any skin ulcers or gangrenous toes?

Do you have problems getting or maintaining erections? (Leriche's syndrome)

Do you have any other vascular diseases? (AAA, angina, previous MI/stroke, peripheral vascular disease in the other leg, renovascular disease)

Are there any symptoms of infection? (Cellulitis, osteomyelitis)

- Fever
- Anorexia

Are there any symptoms of ischaemia?

- Palpitations (emboli)
- Chest pain
- Shortness of breath on exertion
- Syncope
- Skin changes
- Loss of vision
- Speech problems
- Numbness/weakness of limb

Are there any symptoms of DVT?

- Ankle swelling
- Erythema

Neurological associations?

- Muscle weakness
- Wasting
- Sensory problems (feeling as if walking on cotton wool, losing balance when walking in the dark/with eyes closed – painful peripheral neuropathy)
- Bladder or bowel symptoms

Are there any symptoms of a PE?

- Haemoptysis
- Shortness of breath at rest
- Pleuritic chest pain

Precipitating factors

What makes the pain worse? Lifting your legs straight off the bed? Walking?

Is the pain worse going up or down hills/stairs? (Spinal stenosis improves going uphill, unlike vascular disease)

Does cycling or leaning on a Zimmer frame/trolley help or does it make the pain worse? (Relieved in spinal stenosis)

Do you get the pain especially when you stand from sitting, or even just when standing stationary, ie is it truly related to activity?

Is there a history of an infected lesion such as an ingrowing toenail/ boil/ulcerating lesion/insect bite/fungal infection on the feet?

Relieving factors

What helps the pain?

- Resting
- Simple analgesia (NSAIDs)

Does the pain ever wake you from your sleep? Do you sleep with your legs hanging off the bed at night?

How do you sleep? (In a chair?) Does that help?

How long does the pain take to go after you rest? (Vascular pain is relieved quicker by rest, ie after about 1–3 minutes; neurogenic claudication takes longer to recover, about 5–20 minutes)

Severity

How far can you walk? (Flat/incline – stairs/hills)

Does the pain limit you, or does something else?

Can you walk through the pain ever? (Gives an idea of severity and in spinal stenosis patients can never do this)

Where can you walk to? (The local shops?)

Do you ever get the pain at rest?

How far can you walk before the pain starts? Is this getting better/worse/staying the same with time?

Do you have to sit down/lie down to get full relief from pain (spinal stenosis), or will it go away just from stopping walking but still standing up (typical of vascular origin)?

Is the distance to onset of pain constant (vascular) or variable (spinal)?

How bad is the pain?

What effect does it have on your life?

Cardiovascular risk factors – DM, hypertension, high cholesterol, smoking, past history, family history

DVT risk factors – immobility, operations, long flights, OCP, past history of a DVT/PE, family history, hypertension, smoking, pregnancy, dehydration, trauma/casts

---

What do you think is wrong?

Ask about treatment, if any, already received.

➤ Past medical history

Is there any history of previous symptoms/peripheral vascular disease, reconstructive vascular surgery, angioplasties, amputations?

Is there a past history of MIs/strokes/TIAs/chronic lung disease? Have you ever had an irregular heart beat?

Drugs such as aspirin or anticoagulants?

Is there a history of high cholesterol, other vascular disease, DM (how is it controlled?), hypertension?

Do you smoke?

Is there a past history of DVT/PEs, or trauma to the leg?

➤ Drug history

Do you take any medications?

Are you on β-blockers? (Exacerbates claudication)

Compliance, side-effect(s) of medication, OTC/herbal remedies, allergies.

(What happens?)

➤ Social history

Do you smoke? How much? For how long? When did you stop? (Ask if they have tried to stop or congratulate them for stopping)

Do you drink alcohol? How much?

Do you use recreational drugs? (IVDUs and DVT risk)

Have you been abroad? (Overseas travel history, and flights – DVT risk)

Occupation (occupational exposures), exercise capacity, lifestyle limitations due to disease.

Have you taken time off work? How much?

How far can you usually walk and what stops you?

How do the symptoms interfere with your life? (Working, sleeping)

➤ Family history

Is there a family history of malignancy?

Has there been contact with TB or other infections?

Is there a family history of cardiovascular, cerebrovascular, or peripheral vascular disease?

➤ Differential diagnosis

Infection
- **Cellulitis**
- **Osteomyelitis**
- **Septic arthritis**

Neoplasia
- Osteosarcoma
- **Secondary deposits**

Vascular
- **Arterial claudication**
- Acute
  - **Embolic**
  - Dissection
  - Ruptured aneurysm
  - Arteritis
- Chronic (intermittent claudication)
  - **Atherosclerotic**
  - **Thrombotic**
- Venous claudication
  - **Deep vein thrombosis**

Inflammatory/autoimmune
- Vasculitis
- RA
- Seronegative arthritides

Trauma
- **Fractures**
- Haematomas
- Dislocations
- Sprained muscle

Endocrine

- Diabetic complications

Drugs

- **β-Blockers** (exacerbates intermittent claudication)

Metabolic

- Hypocalcaemia (cramps)
- Crystal arthropathy (gout/pseudogout)

Degenerative

- Osteoarthritis
- Ruptured Baker's cyst
- Meniscal lesions

Neurological

- **Neurogenic/spinal claudication**
  - **'Sciatica'** (lumbosacral intervertebral disc prolapse)
  - **Spinal stenosis**
- **Painful peripheral neuropathy**
  - **Diabetes mellitus**
  - **Alcohol**

➤ Investigations

Blood tests

- Haematology – FBC, D-dimers, ESR
    - Anaemia (anaemia of chronic disease)
    - Raised WCC (infection)
    - D-dimers (DVT)
    - ESR (infection, inflammation, malignancy)
- Biochemistry
    - U+Es (CRF, renal involvement in connnective tissue disorder)
    - Ca^{2+} (hypocalcaemic cramps, raised in malignancy)
    - LFTs (alcoholic neuropathy, disseminated malignancy)
    - Glucose (DM → neuropathy, peripheral vascular disease)
    - Lipids (modifiable risk factor for peripheral vascular disease)
    - TFTs (impaired lipid metabolism → peripheral vascular disease)
    - CRP (infection)
    - Serum urate (gout)
- Immunology
    - Autoimmune screen (vasculitis, seronegative arthropathies)
    - Rheumatoid factor (RA)

Microbiology

- Blood cultures (cellulitis, septic arthritis)

ECG

- Arrhythmia (eg AF) → emboli (acutely ischaemic leg)

Urine dipstick

- Glucose (DM)
- Protein, blood (CRF → cramps)

Ankle–brachial pressure index (arterial disease)

Radiology

- Local X-rays
  - Osteoarthritis
  - RA
  - Chondrocalcinosis (pseudogout)
  - Chronic osteomyelitis
  - Osteolysis (tumours)
  - Fractures
  - Foreign body
- USS joint
  - Joint effusion
- Lumbosacral spine X-ray
  - Osteophytes
  - Narrowing of joint spaces
  - Lordosis
- CXR
  - Secondary deposits
- MRI spine (spinal stenosis, sciatica, disc lesions, tumours)
- Duplex Doppler USS (DVT, arterial disease)
- Arteriography – aorta, iliac, femoral, popliteal and distal arteries (vascular disease)

Further investigations

- Venography (DVT)
- Joint aspiration (septic arthritis, gout, pseudogout)
- Nerve conduction studies (nerve lesions, peripheral neuropathy)
- Bone scan

Leg ulcers

➤ History of presenting complaint

Site

Where is the ulcer? (medial/lateral side leg?, foot?)

Onset

Duration?

How was it noticed? (suddenly appeared, painful, itch, bleeding, change in pigmentation etc.).

Character

What is the time course/onset (gradual vs sudden)?

Is it enlarging/staying the same/getting smaller? Over what time course?

Has it quickly got bigger recently (Marjolin's)?

Is it discharging? How deep is it? What lies at it's base? (Tendons? Bones? Slough?)

What colour is it? What is the edge like? (heaped up?)

Radiation

Are there any other ulcers on the body similar to this one?

Associated symptoms

Is it producing local symptoms? Is it **painful or painless?** Does it cause any discomfort?

Do they ache? (When? At the end of the day? After prolonged standing?)

Do your legs swell?

Do you have any:

- Eczema
- Itching
- Pigmentation
- Bruising
- Shiny skin
- Inflammation
- Bleeding

Evidence of ischaemia:

- Do you get pain in your calves when you walk? (claudication)
- Do your feet get cold? Are they pale?
- Do you get pins and needles?
- Do you get any palpitations (emboli)?
- Are you able to feel someone/ something touching your feet?

Malignancy / infective:

- Are there any other symptoms (weight loss, malaise)?
- Have you noticed any abdominal swelling(s)? Have your clothes become tighter recently? (pelvic masses leading to secondary varicose veins – therefore any gynaecological symptoms in females such as increased urinary frequency, urgency, urge incontinence, vaginal bleeding etc.)
- Are there any callosities on your feet suggestive of a neuropathic ulcer?
- Is the ulcer at the site of a previous mole? Is the ulcer pigmented? (malignant melanoma)

Precipitating factors

Is there a history of trauma to the leg?

Do you have varicose veins?

Relieving factors

What do you do to relieve the pain? How do you sleep?

Severity

What problems do they cause?

Does the cosmetic appearance bother you?

Does the pain ever wake you up at night?

> ➤ *Ask about cardiovascular risk factors:*

DM

Hypertension

Smoking

High cholesterol

Past/family history of peripheral vascular disease or amputations

Do you look after your feet?

Do you inspect them regularly?

Do you visit a podiatrist?

What do you think is wrong?

Ask about treatment, if any, already received?

➤ Past medical history

Is there a history of previous illnesses or ulcers? How were previous ulcers managed? Did they heal well? Did they need skin grafting?

Do you wear compression hosiery/stockings?

Is there a past history of DVT/PE, or post phlebetic limb? Have you sustained trauma to the lower limb? (deep venous insufficiency)

Have you had varicose veins in pregnancy? Did one leg swell up in pregnancy? (DVT)

Is there a history of peripheral vascular disease/AF/infective endocarditis (suggests ischaemic ulcers)?

Are you diabetic? Is it well controlled?

Do you suffer from IBD (pyoderma gangrenosum)?

What about RA? Hypertension? Haematological conditions? (All are complicated by ulcers)

Have you had previous surgery for varicosities/peripheral vascular disease/previous amputations? What was done (high tie/strip/multiple avulsions) (ballooning/reconstruction/amputation)? How many operations have been required?

➤ Drug history

Do you take any medications, such as beta-blockers (exacerbates claudication), insulin, anti-hypertensives?

Do you wear stockings?

➤ Social history

Do you smoke? How much and for how long? When did you stop? (Have you tried to stop, or congratulate them for stopping).

Have you been exposed a lot to the sun/got sunburnt?

Occupation (occupational exposures – are you on your feet all day?), exercise capacity, lifestyle limitations due to disease.

➤ Family history

Is there a FHx of amputations or peripheral vascular disease?

Is there a FHx of varicose veins?

Has there been contact with TB or other infections?

Is there a FHx of sickle-cell anaemia?

➤ Differential diagnosis

Venous stasis
- **Deep venous insufficiency**
  - Venous valvular dysfunction
  - Previous DVTs

Arterial/ischaemic
- **Arteriosclerosis**
  - Arteritis
  - Primary vasculitis, eg polyarteritis nodosa
  - Secondary vasculitis, eg RA, SLE
- Arteriovenous fistulae

Neuropathic
- **DM (common)**
- Tabes dorsalis
- Leprosy
- Nerve injuries
- Syringomyelia

Decubitus
- **Pressure (bed sores)**

Malignant
- **Marjolin's ulcer (Squamous cell carcinoma)**
- Melanoma
- Basal cell carcinoma (rare)

Infections
- *Strep. pyogenes*
- Gummatous (syphilis)
- TB

Haematological

- Haemolytic anaemias (sickle cell)
- Polycythaemia rubra vera

Other

- Pyoderma gangrenosum
- Self-inflicted injury:
  - Dermatitis artefacta
- Systemic hypertension (rare)
  - Ulcus hypertensivum (Martorell ulcer)

➤ Investigations

Blood tests

- Haematology – FBC, ESR
  - Hb (haematological disease)
  - Raised WCC (infected ulcer)
  - ESR (vasculitis, syphilis, TB)
- Biochemistry
  - U+Es (renal involvement may suggest autoimmune disease or co-incidental renovascular disease)
  - Glucose and HbA_{1c} (diabetes mellitus)
  - CRP (infection)

Microbiology

- Swab of ulcer (M,C+S)
- VDRL (syphilis serology)

Urine dipstick

- Glucose (DM)

Radiology

- Doppler studies
  - Venous disease
  - Arterial disease

- Local X-ray:
  - Underlying osteomyelitis (chronic)

Ankle–brachial pressure index (arterial disease)

Further investigations

- Rheumatoid factor
- Autoimmune/vasculitic screen (vasculitis/SLE)
- Patch testing (differential diagnosis of venous eczema is contact dermatitis)
- Biopsy (Marjolin's ulcer)
- Angiography (definitive diagnosis of peripheral vascular disease)
- Venography (assess varicose veins, deep venous patency)
- Hb electrophoresis, blood film (sickle cell)

Lower gastrointestinal bleeding

➤ History of presenting complaint

Onset

When did it start?

Have you ever had this before, or is this a new symptom?

Was it sudden and spontaneous?

How often does it occur during the day?

Does it stop spontaneously?

Character

Composition of bleed – fresh red, dark or melaena ('tarry')? Clots or liquid?

Is it fresh red blood, mixed in with the stool, or melaena? Does it smell pungent?

Does it drip into the pan?

Is it on the toilet paper?

Does it coat the surface of the stool?

How much blood is there per motion? (Diverticular disease, angiodysplasia may be massive, but latter often causes repeated, small bleeds)

Did you notice the blood only on one occasion or on many? Is it continuous and every time you pass stool, or intermittent?

Does it only occur with defecation, or does it necessitate wearing something like a pad if it occurs all the time?

Radiation

Is there a recent history of epistaxis or haemoptysis with swallowed blood?

Do blood or faeces stain your underwear at all?

Associated symptoms

Are there any symptoms of shock, such as dizziness upon standing, palpitations, etc?

Is there any nausea, vomiting, haematemesis or bleeding elsewhere?

Is there any mucus/pus in the stool?

Have you had a change in bowel habit?

Is there any diarrhoea? (Nocturnal as in UC) Constipation? What is normal for you?

Do you have any itching around the back passage, or the sensation of something coming down when you pass stool? (Haemorrhoids, rectal prolapse)

Do you have the feeling of a lump in the anus? (Solitary rectal ulcer)

Is it associated with any **pain**? (Anal fissure, diverticular disease, carcinoma of the anal canal, ischaemic colitis, perianal Crohn's disease) Is the pain continuous or brought on by defecation? Is it colicky? Is it brought on by food? (Mesenteric angina)

Is there any tenesmus? (Feeling that the bowels are not empty despite defecation) Is there urgency?

Are there any systemic features? (Weight loss, fever, arthralgia, skin changes, eye changes/pain)

Are there symptoms of a UTI (colovaginal fistulae), dirty urine, pneumaturia?

Precipitating factors

What precipitated the bleed?

Was it precipitated by passing stool? (After/during or before passing a motion; haemorrhoids typically bleed after a motion)

Is there a history of trauma to the anal canal or a history of abuse?

What do you think is wrong?

Ask about treatment, if any, already received.

➤ Past medical history

Is there a history of previous illnesses, such as UC, carcinoma bowel, diverticular disease or bleeding PUD?

Have any polyps been removed from your bowels in the past?

Is there a history of haemorrhoids or anal fissure?

Do you have any bleeding disorders? Do you bruise spontaneously? Do you bleed from any other sites?

Is there a history of radiotherapy? (Carcinoma cervix – irradiation proctitis/colitis)

Is there a history of heart disease? (Mesenteric infarction)

Have you had any infections in the bowel recently?

Have you had any recent surgery or colonoscopies? (AAA repair?)

Have you ever had a barium enema?

➤ Drug history

Are you taking any anticoagulants?

Are you on iron tablets?

Do you take lots of anti-inflammatories? (Collagenous colitis)

Do you take bismuth? (Black stool, like iron and not red)

Have you had any recent courses of antibiotics?

Compliance, side-effect(s) of medication, OTC/herbal remedies, allergies.

(What happens?)

➤ Social history

Do you smoke? How much?

Do you consume much alcohol?

Have you been abroad? (Overseas travel history, tropical illnesses)

Have you taken time off work? How much?

› Family history

Is there a family history of carcinoma bowel, polyps, IBD?

› Differential diagnosis

General

Bleeding diastheses – anticoagulation therapy, haemophilia, etc.

Local

Anal

- **Haemorrhoids**
- **Anal fissure**
- **Carcinoma**
- Trauma

Rectum and descending colon

- **Colonic carcinoma and polyps**
- **Diverticular bleed**
- **Colitis**
    - **Ulcerative**
    - **Crohn's**
    - **Ischaemic**
    - **Pseudomembranous**
    - **Infective** (*Campylobacter*, haemorrhagic *Escherichia coli*, *Salmonella*, *Shigella*, *Clostridium*, amoebic dysentery all cause bloody diarrhoea)
    - Microscopic
    - Collagenous
    - Lymphocytic/eosinophilic
- Irradiation colitis/proctitis
- Solitary rectal ulcer

Caecum/ascending colon

- **Caecal/colonic carcinoma and polyps**
- **Angiodysplasia**
- **Mesenteric infarction**
- Meckel's diverticulum

Upper GI bleeds

- Invariably melaena unless very large upper GI bleed (eg DU, aorto-enteric fistula)

Differentiation of diverticular disease from carcinoma of the colon can sometimes be difficult. The following table may help:

	Diverticular disease	Carcinoma
History	Long	Short
Pain	More common	25% painless
Mass	25% have tenderness	Non-tender
Bleeding	17%; often profuse, periodic, without warning	65%; usually small amounts and persistent
Radiograph	Diffuse change and presence of diverticula	Localised, short segment of bowel
	Gradual transition from normal to diseased bowel	Abrupt transition
	Strictures have tapered ends and smooth outline	Strictures have shouldered edges and an irregular lumen ('apple-core configuration')
	Spasticity may be relieved	No relaxation with propantheline bromide
	Mucosa normally intact and saw-tooth pattern may be seen	Destruction of the mucosal folds
Sigmoidoscopy	Inflammatory change over an area	No inflammation until ulcer is reached
Colonoscopy	No carcinoma seen	Carcinoma seen and can be biopsied

> Investigations

Blood tests

- Haematology – FBC, clotting, ESR, cross-match/G+S
  - Anaemia (severe bleeding, malignancy, chronic colitis)
  - WCC (IBD, ischaemic colitis, infective colitis)
  - Thrombocytopenia (bleeding diathesis)
  - Clotting/INR (bleeding diathesis causing/aggravating bleeding)
  - ESR (carcinoma, IBD, vasculitis (PAN))
  - Cross match/G+S (severe bleed)
- Biochemistry
  - U+Es (urea disproportionately high due to blood absorption)
  - LFTs (liver failure and oesophageal varices, metastases)
  - CRP (infection)
  - Cardiac enzymes – troponin I/T (MI)
  - Tumour markers, eg CEA (tumour of GI tract)

Faecal occult blood

Microbiology

- Blood cultures (infective cause of bloody diarrhoea)
- Stool culture (organisms in infective cause, WCC in IBD, *Clostridium difficile* toxin)

ECG

- AF → embolic mesenteric infarct
- (Old) MI → mesenteric ischaemia
- Cardiac ischaemia if massive blood loss

Arterial blood gases

- Lactic acidosis (bowel ischaemia/infarct)

Radiology

- AXR
  - Obstruction associated with neoplasm
  - Toxic megacolon (IBD)
  - Barium enema
  - Polps/carcinoma
  - Diverticular disease
  - IBD
  - Ischaemic colitis
- Liver USS
  - Metastases
- CT thorax, abdomen, pelvis
  - Staging of carcinoma

Endoscopy

- Proctoscopy/sigmoidoscopy ± biopsy
  - Ano-rectal tumours
  - Haemorrhoids
  - Distal colitis/proctitis
- Colonoscopy ± biopsy
  - Diverticular disease
  - Polyps/colonic tumours
  - Angiodysplasia
  - Colitis
- OGD ± biopsy (upper GI bleed)

Further investigations

- Mesenteric angiography (actively bleeding angiodysplasia, Meckel's diverticulum, ischaemic colitis)
- Labelled red cell scan (angiodysplasia, Meckel's diverticulum)
- Technetium scan (Meckel's diverticulum)
- Small-bowel follow-through (small-bowel tumours)
- Surgical exploration

Lumps (general)

See also sections on Breast lump, Neck lumps and Lymphadenopathy.

➤ History of presenting complaint

Site

Where is the lump?

Onset

How was it noticed? (Gradual vs sudden onset – if acute, think about infections, trauma, haematomas)

Is it enlarging/staying the same/getting smaller? Over what time course?

Character

Any changes in size, shape and colour? (Change in pigmentation, etc)

Associated symptoms

Pain, itch, bleeding, discomfort, discharge, redness, heat?

Timing

Duration.

Predisposing factors

Sun, insect bite, trauma, infection, etc.

Other

Are there other lumps on the body similar to this one?

Systemic symptoms

Are there any other symptoms? (Fever, weight loss, rigors (severe shaking episodes), malaise)

What do you think is wrong?

Ask about treatment if any, already received or suggested.

➤ Past medical history

MITJTHREADS

Is there a history of previous illnesses, or other lumps?

➤ Drug history

Do you take any medications?

Compliance, side-effect(s) of medication, OTC/herbal remedies, allergies. (What happens?)

➤ Social history

Have you been abroad? (Overseas travel history, tropical illnesses)

Occupation (occupational exposures), exercise capacity, lifestyle limitations due to disease.

➤ Family history

Is there a family history of malignancy?

Has there been contact with a person with TB or any other infection?

Is there a family history of multiple lipomas? (Dercum's disease or adiposis dolorosa)

Lumps (general)

➤ Differential diagnosis

Skin

- **Sebaceous cyst**
- **Lipoma**
- Haematoma
- Sarcoma
- Skin tag
- Dermoid cyst
- **Ganglion**

Breast

- **Carcinoma**
- **Fibroadenoma**
- **Fibroadenosis**
- Fat necrosis
- Galactocele
- Duct ectasia
- Abscess

Abdomen

Right hypochondrium	Epigastric	Left hypochondrium

Hepatomegaly
Empyema of gallbladder
Mucocele of gallbladder
	Gastric carcinoma
	Abdominal aortic aneurysm
	Pancreatic mass:
	  carcinoma
	  pseudocyst
		Splenomegaly

Right loin/flank	**Central/periumbilical**	**Left loin/flank**
Enlarged kidney	Pancreatic carcinoma **Abdominal aortic aneurysm**	**Enlarged kidney**
Right iliac fossa	**Suprapubic**	**Left iliac fossa**
Caecal carcinoma **Crohn's disease** **Appendiceal abscess** Ileocaecal TB Lymphadenopathy **Transplanted pelvic kidney** **Large ovarian cyst/ tumour**	**Enlarged bladder** Pregnancy **Fibroids**	Constipation **Colonic cancer** **Diverticular abscess** Lymphadenopathy **Transplanted pelvic kidney** **Large ovarian cyst/ tumour**

Inguinal

- **Direct/indirect inguinal hernia**
- **Femoral hernia**
- **Lymphadenopathy**
- Saphena varix
- **Femoral artery aneurysm** (true or false)
- **Undescended testis**

Scrotal

- **Indirect inguinal hernia**
- **Hydrocele**
- Epididymal cyst
- Haematocele
- **Testicular tumour**
- Orchitis (mumps)
- Tuberculous epididymitis

➤ Investigations

Radiology

- USS
  - Defines location, origin and extent of lump
  - Determines size of lump
  - Solid vs cystic/multicystic (hetero/homogeneity)
  - Solitary vs multiple lumps
- CT
  - Defines local anatomy
  - Relationship of lump to adjacent structures
  - Staging for malignancy

Further investigations

Depend on site, clinical findings and radiology.

Lymphadenopathy (general)

➤ History of presenting complaint

Site

Which glands have been noticed as enlarged and by whom? (Generalised vs local lymphadenopathy)

For how long?

Onset

When did it start?

Character

Are they still increasing in size?

Have they enlarged before? (Fluctuating changes in size are typical of lymphoma)

Are they painful/tender? Soft/hard?

Is there disfigurement or do they rub against your clothes?

Associated symptoms

Are there any associated symptoms?

- Weight loss
- Fever (character – Pel–Ebstein)
- Night sweats
- Anorexia
- Malaise
- Pruritus
- Alcohol-induced pain
- Cough
- Sputum
- Haemoptysis
- Sore throat/tonsillitis
- Rash/erythema (eg cellulitis, rubella, SLE, sarcoid)

- Change in voice (EBV, recurrent laryngeal nerve involvement in malignancy)
- Arthralgia/arthropathy (infective cause)
- Back pain

Are there any other lumps/masses on the body? (Such as breast, thyroid carcinoma spread to cervical lymph nodes)

Are there any other symptoms of primary carcinomas – shortness of breath, cough, dysphagia, dyspepsia, hoarseness, nasal discharge, deafness? (Carcinoma lung/oesophagus/stomach/larynx/thyroid/nasopharynx all spread to cervical lymph nodes)

Are other family members fit and well?

Are there any symptoms of thyrotoxicosis – heat intolerance, weight loss, diarrhoea, tremor, increased appetite, irritability?

Precipitating factors

Is there a history of local trauma?

Has there been any contact with glandular fever, TB, or any other infections?

Have you been scratched by any cats recently?

What do you think is wrong?

Ask about treatment, if any, already received.

➤ Past medical history

Is there a history of previous illnesses? (SLE, RA, sarcoid)

Is there a history of malignancy, TB, travel?

Is there a past history of head and neck cancer?

Have you been a recipient of any blood transfusions/products? (HIV risk)

➤ Drug history

Do you take any medications, especially phenytoin, allopurinol?

Have you been in contact with beryllium?

Compliance, side-effect(s) of medication, OTC/herbal remedies, allergies. (What happens?)

➤ Social history

Do you use or have you ever used recreational drugs? (HIV risk)

Have you been abroad? (Overseas travel history, tropical illnesses) Do you remember being bitten by an insect? (Lyme disease, ehrlichiosis)

Do you keep animals at home? Cats or dogs (cat-scratch disease, toxoplasmosis)?

Occupation (occupational exposures).

Sexual history required – HIV risk:

- Have you had unprotected sex? (Inguinal lymph nodes – HSV, *lymphogranuloma venereum*)
- 'I need to ask you some important but rather personal questions':
  - (Men) Have you ever had sex with another man?
  - (Woman) Have you ever had sex with a man known to be bisexual?
- Is there any chance that you may be pregnant? (If not, advise the patient strongly not to become pregnant under any circumstances as toxoplasmosis and CMV, which are both causes of lymphadenopathy, are potentially teratogenic)
- Have all your partners been from the UK?
- Have you received or donated blood products?
- Have you ever had an HIV test?
- Have you been in contact with anyone who has injected drugs?

➤ Family history

Is there a family history of malignancy?

Have you been in contact with anyone with TB, glandular fever or other infections?

➤ Differential diagnosis

Localised

Infective

- Acute infection
  - Viral
    - ➤ EBV
    - ➤ CMV
    - ➤ Measles
    - ➤ Rubella
  - Bacterial
    - ➤ Cat-scratch disease
  - Protozoal
    - ➤ Toxoplasmosis
- Chronic infection
  - TB
  - HIV
- Secondary infection
  - Secondary to local infection/inflammation (eg tonsillitis), infected skin lesion (eg infected sebaceous cyst), or local abscess

Neoplastic

- Primary – lymphoma (Hodgkin's)
- Secondary spread of tumour from local site

Generalised causes of lymphadenopathy

Infective

- Acute
  - EBV
  - CMV
  - Sepsis
- Chronic
  - HIV
  - TB

- Brucellosis
- Secondary syphilis

Neoplastic

- Lymphoma
  - Hodgkin's
  - Non-Hodgkin's
- Leukaemias
  - Acute lymphocytic leukaemia
  - Chronic lymphocytic leukaemia

Inflammatory

- SLE
- Sarcoidosis
- RA
- Berylliosis

Drugs (pseudolymphoma)

- Phenytoin
- Allopurinol
- Sulphonamides

Rare causes

- Dermatopathic lymphadenopathy
  - Psoriasis
  - Eczema
- Thyrotoxicosis
- Sinus histiocytosis
- IVDU

- Lipoidoses (eg Gaucher's, Niemann–Pick)
- Kimura's disease
- Whipple's disease
- Kikuchi's disease

> Investigations

Blood tests
- Haematology – FBC, clotting, ESR, blood film
  - Anaemia (blood dyscrasias)
  - Raised WCC (leukaemia, infection)
  - Differential WCC (leukaemia)
  - Clotting (blood dyscrasias)
  - Raised ESR (infection, lymphoma, malignancy, sarcoidosis)
  - Blood film (leukaemia, reactive)
- Biochemistry
  - U+Es (renal function)
  - CRP (infection)
  - LFTs (malignant infiltration of liver)
  - Uric acid (raised in lymphoma)
  - Serum ACE (sarcoidosis)
  - TFTs (thyrotoxicosis)
- Virology
  - HIV, EBV, measles, CMV, rubella serology
  - Paul–Bunnell/Monospot test (EBV)
- Immunology
  - Antibody screen (SLE, RA)
  - Toxoplasmosis antibody titres
  - Lyme serology
  - VDRL (syphilis)

Microbiology
- Blood cultures (TB, brucellosis, sepsis)
- Swab (local infections)
- Mantoux/Heaf test (TB)

Radiology

- CXR
  - Hilar lymphadenopathy (sarcoidosis, lymphoma)
  - Carcinoma (primary or secondaries)
  - TB
- USS ± FNAC lymph node (malignancy)
- CT thorax, abdomen, pelvis
  - Defines mass in relation to anatomical neighbours
  - Nodal distribution
  - Staging of Hodgkin's

Further investigations

- Lymph node biopsy
- Bone marrow aspirate/trephine biopsy (lymphoma, leukaemia)
- Other investigations to locate source of potential primary carcinoma:
  - Mammography (breast carcinoma)
  - Laryngoscopy (laryngeal carcinoma)
  - Panendoscopy (nasopharyngeal, oropharyngeal, laryngopharyngeal carcinoma)
  - OGD (oesophageal or gastric carcinoma)
  - Bronchoscopy (lung carcinoma)

Multiply injured patient

➤ History of presenting complaint

Any history that is obtained is a valuable part of the secondary survey of advanced trauma life support (ATLS) management, but to be able to extract the **most important** features of the history as part of a **rapid** patient assessment in a resuscitation setting requires the use of an **AMPLE** history:

> **A**llergies
>
> **M**edications (current)
>
> **P**MHx, **P**regnancy status
>
> **L**ast meal – timing (general anaesthetic risk), **L**ast tetanus
>
> **E**vents and **E**nvironment surrounding the accident (mechanism of injury)

*For **all** trauma situations ask about:*

What happened/circumstances of injury?

How did it occur?

What is the likelihood of other associated injuries?

What time did the accident occur?

How much time has elapsed since the injury?

Eliciting the exact mechanism of injury will provide a valuable impression of the nature of the forces involved (and therefore the severity of injuries sustained) and the likelihood of associated injuries and subsequent complications. Try to gather information from other witnesses, friends/family, paramedics, police etc.

For an RTA try to elicit the exact mechanism of injury:

What type of vehicle were you travelling in? (Car/motorbike/HGV/PSV, make of vehicle, etc)

Were any passengers with you in your vehicle when the accident took place? How many? What about children?

Where were you sitting in the vehicle? (Were you the driver or a passenger?)

Do you remember anything about the accident or events preceding/leading up to the accident? (Retrograde amnesia)

Have you been able to remember what has happened since the accident? (Anterograde amnesia)

What caused the accident? How fast were you going? How fast was the other vehicle going? What sort of road were you on? (Motorway, A road, B road, 1/2/3/4-lane road? Was there a central reservation? Was there a hard shoulder?) Which lane were you in?

Mode of impact

What did you hit? (Another car, a bike, a stationary object, a pedestrian, ie Did you hit a mobile or immovable object?)

Was the other car going in the same direction as you, perpendicular to you, or in the opposite direction to you when you collided?

Which part of your car was hit? (Front, back, passenger side, driver side)

Did you or the other vehicle slow down at all before you collided?

Did you **lose consciousness** during the accident? If so, was it at the moment of impact or afterwards?

How long did you lose consciousness for? (Seconds, minutes, hours or days)

Were the other passengers badly injured or killed in the accident? Did they lose consciousness?

Did you hit any part of your body on the dashboard when you collided?

If children were involved in the crash, did they cry immediately (a normal response) or were they limp and unresponsive?

Post-RTA

What state was your vehicle in after impact?

What about the object/vehicle you hit?

Was the windshield smashed? Was the car a 'write off'? Was there significant intrusion into the driver/passenger compartments?

What position were you and the passengers in after the collision?

Was anyone trapped in the vehicle? How long for?

Precipitating factors

What caused you to crash/lose control of the wheel in the first place?

What happened immediately prior to the accident?

Had you had anything to drink before you set out?

Did you use any street drugs prior to setting out?

Did you have any chest pain or fitting at the time of the accident?

Are you diabetic? Were your blood sugar levels low prior to setting out on your journey?

Do you suffer from poor vision?

Were you tired at the wheel or had you been driving for a long period of time without an adequate rest period?

What were the driving conditions like at the time of impact? (Night, foggy, snow, windy, ice, raining, frost, spray from road, etc) Were your headlights working? What about the other vehicle?

Provision and use of safety features

Do you have an airbag on your car? What about a passenger airbag? Did either or both inflate/deploy? Did you sustain any injuries (eg to your eye) as a result of airbag insufflation?

Is your car fitted with seatbelts? What about rear seatbelts? Were you wearing a seatbelt at the time? Were your passengers?

Does your car have headrests? For whom? Does your car possess side-impact bars?

For (motor)cyclists, were you wearing a crash helmet at the time of impact?

For all other (non-RTA) injuries

How did you sustain the injury?

Was the object sharp or blunt?

How deep did it penetrate? (mm, cm)

Who caused the injury? Do you have a safe home to go to?

How far did you fall?

What sort of surface did you fall on to? (Grass, concrete, etc)

Where did it occur? (Contaminated or clean environment?)

Do you have pain/tenderness? (At night? Pinpoint tenderness?) Where?

Has there been sudden loss of function of the part that you injured?

Is there deformity?

Is there swelling, discoloration or bruising?

What position was your hand in when you fell?

Why did you fall?

Did you just trip or was there something more to it?

Did you lose consciousness during the episode? Was there any chest pain preceding the fall? Was there any tongue biting or urinary incontinence?

(See Collapse, syncope and blackouts)

Fractures

*In taking the history of a patient who may have a **fracture**, the following questions may prove helpful:*

What activity was being pursued at the time of the incident?

What was the nature of the incident?

What was the magnitude of the applied forced? (For example, for a fall from a height it is helpful to know the distance fallen, if the fall was broken, the manner of the landing and the nature of the surface on which the patient landed)

Where on the body was the point of impact and the direction of the applied forces?

Is there any significance to be attached to the incident itself? (For example, if there was a fall, was it precipitated by some underlying medical condition such as a hypotensive attack which requires separate investigation?)

Where is the site of any pain, and what is its severity?

Is there loss of functional activity? (For example, walking is seldom possible after any fracture of the tibia or femur; inability to weight-bear after an incident is of great significance)

Burns

For burns, specifically ask:

Was the injury sustained by accident, or was it an act of deliberate self-harm/attempted suicide?

What did you burn yourself with?

- Thermal burns
  - Fire
  - Boiling water
  - Steam
  - Gas
  - Cold
  - Sun
- Chemical burn
- Radiation burn
- Electrical burn

Nature of the burning agent involved? (Furniture, steam, petrol, gas etc – some burning substances such as polyvinyl chloride can give off toxic fumes such as cyanides)

Is there any pain? Is there swelling and blistering?

Was there an explosion? Was there a warning first? (Such as a smoke alarm)

Where were you when it took place – were you at home or at work?

Did you inhale any smoke?

Was the fire in an enclosed space? (Risk of carbon monoxide poisoning)

When did the fire start? (Timing is important for later fluid management)

When were you removed from the fire?

How long were you exposed for?

What clothing were you wearing at the time?

Do you suffer from impaired sensation, eg diabetes? Were/are you able to feel the burn?

Was first aid instituted and cold water applied?

Was there a history of confusion/loss of consciousness/fainting surrounding the incident? (Alcoholism, IVDUs, epilepsy)

Did you hit your head on the way down?

Associated injuries

Blood loss – Are you bleeding from anywhere? (**Overt** haemorrhage)

Do you feel dizzy at all when you stand up from the sitting or lying position? (**Covert/concealed** haemorrhage)

Cervical spine integrity

Do you have any neck pain or numbness?

Do you have any pins and needles, or numbness down your arms, or in your hands?

Have you had any previous whiplash injuries?

NB: Any patient with a blunt injury sustained above the level of the clavicles has a cervical spine injury until proved otherwise.

Head injury (haematoma)

- Drowsiness/difficulty rousing
- Confusion
- Headaches (Is it worsening?)
- Dizziness
- Loss of balance
- Nausea and vomiting
- Double vision/blurred vision
- Visual disturbances
- Fitting/seizures
- Slurred speech
- Limb weakness
- Sensory disturbances – numbness/pins and needles
- Personality changes
- Hearing

Do you have any amnesia/memory loss? (Anterograde amnesia – for the events that followed the incident – vs retrograde amnesia – events that led up to the incident)

Do you have any ear or nasal discharge? (CSF otorrhoea/rhinorrhoea)

Do you have normal bladder and bowel function? (Retention/incontinence)

For children – Has there been a change in the child's normal behaviour?

Chest

Tension/open pneumothorax, aortic rupture, haemothorax, tamponade, flail chest, inhalational injury, bone/back/rib pain (fractures) – *ask*:

Is there any chest pain? Is it worse on breathing?

Is there any shortness of breath?

Do you have difficulty breathing?

Do you have a hoarse voice?

Abdomen

Do you have any abdominal pain or distension?

Do you have any shoulder-tip pain? (Splenic rupture)

Have you noticed any blood in your urine? (Kidney)

Do you have normal bladder and bowel function?

Ask about pre-hospital care, if any, already received.

➤ Past medical history

Is there a history of previous orthopaedic/trauma operations?

Ask if there is a history of any significant/pre-existing medical conditions, including:

- Cardiorespiratory compromise
- Epilepsy, diabetes

What about bleeding disorders?

Previous head or other orthopaedic injuries? (Would make X-rays confusing)

➤ Drug history

Do you take any medications?

- Anticoagulants
- Immunosuppressants

Is your tetanus immunisation up to date? When was your last tetanus booster?

➤ Social history

Alcohol intake – drink driving?

Use of recreational drugs.

What was the pre-morbid state of the patient?

What is your occupation? Will you still be able to do this?

Is there someone at home with you? Will they be able to manage?

Do you have a telephone at home in case you become poorly?

➤ Investigations

Blood tests

- Haematology – FBC, clotting, cross-match/G+S
  - Anaemia (bleeding)
  - Haematocrit (bleeding, burns)
  - Clotting (bleeding)
  - Cross-match/G+S (severe bleed)
- Biochemistry
  - U+Es (renal function)
  - Glucose
  - LFTs (liver function)
  - Carboxyhaemoglobin levels (burns)
- Arterial blood gases (lung function)

Multiply injured patient

Microbiology

- Swab of burn/wounds

ECG

- ± cardiac enzymes, especially for electrical burns

Urinalysis

- Blood (renal trauma)
- Myoglobinuria

Radiology

- First-line (before secondary survey begins)
  - Lateral cross-table cervical spine X-ray (fracture, disruption)
  - Pelvic X-ray (AP supine) (fracture)
  - CXR (AP supine)
    - ➤ Haemothorax
    - ➤ Tension/open pneumothorax
    - ➤ Dissection/aortic rupture (widened mediastinum)
    - ➤ Rib fractures (flail chest, associated abdominal trauma if fractured lower ribs)
    - ➤ Inhalational injury
    - ➤ Diaphragmatic tear
    - ➤ Pneumomediastinum (oesophageal rupture)
    - ➤ Subcutaneous/surgical emphysema
    - ➤ Pulmonary contusion
- After secondary survey
  - Skull X-ray (fracture)
  - Abdominal X-ray
  - X-ray long bones (fracture)
  - Abdominal USS (blood)
  - Echocardiography
    - ➤ Cardiac tamponade
  - CT head
    - ➤ Haematoma
  - CT abdomen
    - ➤ Visceral injury

Further investigations

- Toxicology (plasma, urine, gastric aspirate)
- Diagnostic peritoneal lavage
- Laparoscopy

Neck lumps

See also Lymphadenopathy (general).

➤ History of presenting complaint

Site

Where is the lump?

Onset

Duration?

Gradual or sudden?

How was it noticed? (Suddenly, painful, itch, bleeding, change in colour)

Character

Single or multiple?

Hard or soft?

Does it gurgle? (Pharyngeal pouch)

Time course

Is it enlarging/staying the same/getting smaller with time?

Associated symptoms

Are there any local symptoms – pain, redness, tenderness, discharge, heat, stridor/respiratory distress, hoarse voice, dysphagia, gurgling?

Are there any local lesions – mouth decay, mouth ulcers, lumps in mouth/throat/nose/ear, pain/discharge from nose/ears, enlarged tonsils, sore throat?

Other

Are there any other lumps, eg head, face, breasts, testicles? (Carcinoma spread)

Exacerbating factors

Sight of food/mastication, after eating?

Do you get bouts of coughing/choking when lying down, or do you aspirate at all?

Systemic symptoms

Have you had any recent viral illnesses or been feeling feverish? Have you been in contact with anyone who has been ill?

Do you get any blackouts or dizziness? (Chemodectoma)

Does the lump pulsate? (Carotid tumour, aneurysm, ectatic carotid)

Do you get pins and needles or numbness in your hands? Is there wasting of the hand muscles? Do your hands feel abnormally cold? (Cervical rib)

Do you have fever, itching, night sweats, loss of appetite, malaise? Have you lost weight?

Thyroid function

Are there any features of thyroid dysfunction? (Double vision, painful red eyes, weight loss/gain, tremor, palpitations, sweating, hot/cold intolerance, constipation/diarrhoea, heavy periods, hirsutism, hoarse voice, skin changes, alteration in mental functioning)

Movements

Does the lump move, eg when you stick out your tongue or swallow?

What do you think is wrong?

Ask about treatment, if any, already received.

➤ Past medical history

MITJTHREADS

Is there a history of previous illnesses or of other lumps?

Have you had TB or malignancy?

Do you get recurrent chest infections?

Have you been exposed to radiation or radiotherapy?

Have you been a recipient of blood products/transfusions? (HIV risk)

➤ Drug history

Do you take any medications? (Phenytoin, allopurinol – both drugs cause lymphadenopathy)

Lithium treatment? (Goitre)

➤ Social history

Do you use recreational drugs? (HIV)

Have you been abroad? (Overseas travel history, tropical illnesses)

Ethnicity? (TB)

Have you been in contact with animals? Have you been scratched by any cats?

Occupation (eg glass-blowers and laryngoceles; occupational exposures, such as radiotherapy), exercise capacity, lifestyle limitations due to disease?

How do the symptoms interfere with your life? (Walking, working, sleeping)

Have you had unprotected sex? (HIV)

➤ Family history

Is there a family history of malignancy?

Have you been in contact with anyone with TB or any other infections?

➤ Differential diagnosis

Multiple lumps

- **Lymph nodes** (invariably)
- Cold abscess (TB, actinomycosis)

Single lumps

- Superficial
  - **Sebaceous cyst**
  - **Lipoma**
  - Dermoid cyst
  - Abscess
- Deep

	Anterior triangle	Posterior triangle
Does not move with swallowing	Submandibular swelling **Parotid swelling** **Branchial cyst** Carotid body tumour Carotid artery aneurysm Sternomastoid 'tumour' Lymph node/cold abscess Laryngocele Chondroma	Cystic hygroma (lymphangioma) Pharyngeal pouch Cervical rib Subclavian artery aneurysm Tumour of clavicle Lymph node/cold abscess
Moves with swallowing	**Thyroglossal cyst** **Thyroid gland (see below)** Thyroid isthmus lymph node	

Thyroid swellings

- Diffuse, homogeneous enlargement
  - Simple hyperplastic 'physiological' goitre (puberty, menstruation, pregnancy, dietary)
  - **Graves' goitre**
  - **Multinodular goitre** (Plummer's syndrome)
  - Thyroiditis (**Hashimoto's**, de Quervain's or Riedel's)
  - Drug-induced goitre (lithium, amiodarone, antithyroid drugs)
  - Infiltration (sarcoid, amyloid)

Neck lumps

- Solitary nodule
  - **Dominant nodule of a multinodular goitre**
  - Haemorrhage into a nodule
  - Adenoma
  - Simple thyroid cyst
  - **Carcinoma** – primary (papillary, follicular, anaplastic, medullary, lymphoma) or secondary (rare)
  - Enlargement of the whole of one lobe (usually Hashimoto's disease)

➤ Investigations

Blood tests
- Haematology – FBC, ESR, blood film
  - Anaemia (malignancy)
  - Raised WCC (leukaemia, infection)
  - Differential WCC (leukaemia)
  - Raised ESR (infection, lymphoma, malignancy, sarcoidosis)
  - Blood film (leukaemia/lymphoma, reactive)
- Biochemistry
  - U+Es (renal function)
  - TFTs (goitre)
  - LFTs (hepatic involvement in leukaemia, lymphoma)
  - CRP (infection)
  - Uric acid (raised in lymphoma)
  - Serum ACE (sarcoidosis)
  - Cholesterol (raised in myxoedema)
- Virology
  - Viral titres – HIV, EBV, CMV serology
  - Paul–Bunnell/Monospot test (EBV)
- Immunology
  - Thyroid autoantibodies (antiperoxidase (previously called antimicrosomal), antithyroglobulin, TSH receptor antibodies)

Microbiology

- Blood cultures (TB, brucellosis)
- Toxoplasmosis antibody titres
- Mantoux/Heaf test (TB)
- Lyme serology

ECG

- AF (thyrotoxicosis)

Radiology

- Floor of mouth X-ray – salivary calculus
- CXR
  - Hilar lymphadenopathy (sarcoidosis, lymphoma)
  - TB
  - Tumour (primary or secondary)
  - Tracheal deviation (thyroid swelling)
  - Cervical rib
- USS ± FNAC (lymph nodes, thyroid, salivary glands)
- CT lump
  - Defines mass in relation to anatomical neighbours
- CT thorax, abdomen, pelvis
  - Staging

Further investigations

- Bone marrow aspirate/trephine biopsy (lymphoma, leukaemia)
- Lymph node biopsy (lymphoma)
- Thyroid uptake scans
- Sialogram (calculus, stricture)
- Barium swallow (pharyngeal pouch)
- Duplex Doppler
  - Carotid artery aneurysm
  - Ectatic carotid artery
  - Chemodectoma
  - Subclavian artery aneurysm

- Other investigations to locate source of potential primary carcinoma:
  - Mammography (breast carcinoma)
  - Laryngoscopy (laryngeal carcinoma)
  - Panendoscopy (nasopharyngeal, oropharyngeal, laryngopharyngeal carcinoma, other SCC tumours of the head and neck)
  - OGD (oesophageal or gastric carcinoma)
  - Bronchoscopy (lung carcinoma)

Nipple discharge

➤ History of presenting complaint

Site

Is it from the left breast, right breast or both?

Onset

Duration? How was it noticed?

Character

Character (milky, serous, green, brown, yellow, bloody)?

Is it frank red blood, or altered blood (darkish brown)?

Has it changed in character over time?

Is the discharge produced spontaneously or only when pressure is put on the nipple?

Is it coming from one nipple or both?

Is it coming from one duct or multiple ducts? (former more sinister)

Have you breast-fed recently (in the last year)? (discharge is significant if it continues > 1 year after stopping breast-feeding)

Associated symptoms

Are there any underlying breast lumps or general lumpiness?

Are there any skin changes – eczema, ulceration, retraction, discoloration/pigmentation, tethering?

Are there any nipple changes – inversion, puckering etc?

Is there any breast pain?

Are there any other symptoms – swollen glands, fever, other lumps, weight loss, back pain, breathlessness, swollen arms.

Precipitating factors

Is there any variation with the menstrual cycle?

Is there any possibility that you could be pregnant (and the discharge physiological)?

When was the first day of your LMP?

Are there any features of a prolactinoma – amenorrhoea, infertility, loss of libido, visual changes, headaches etc?

Severity

Quantity – How many times do you have to change your bra each day?

What do you think is wrong?

Concerns (carcinoma)/ideas/expectations.

Ask about treatment, if any, already received?

➤ Past medical history

Is there a history of previous illnesses or other breast lumps? If so what treatment did you receive? (eg mastectomies, wide local excision, radiotherapy, chemotherapy, breast reconstruction, other operations).

Is there a history of other serious illnesses? (carcinoma)

Tell me about your pregnancy history? How many children do you have and when?

Did you breast-feed them?

When did your periods start and finish? (menarche/menopause)

Do you use or have you used the OCP and/or HRT?

➤ Drug history

Do you take any medications such as:

- Antidopaminergic drugs (hyperprolactinaemia)
- Oestrogens or tamoxifen

Have you ever undergone a course of chemotherapy?

Do you use, or have you ever used, the OCP or HRT? How long for?

> Social history

Do you smoke? How much and for how long? When did you stop?

> Family history

Is there a FHx of malignancy, especially breast or ovarian cancers?

> Differential diagnosis

Bloodstained

- **Intraductal papilloma** (discharge from **one** duct)
- **Intraductal carcinoma** (discharge from **one** duct)
- **Duct ectasia** (discharge usually from **multiple** ducts)
- Paget's disease of nipple
- Invasive carcinoma (unusual)

Serous

- Early pregnancy

Yellow/brown/green

- Duct ectasia
- Fibrocystic disease

Milky

- Galactorrhoea
  - Physiological: lactation, late pregnancy, lactation in newborn/puberty
  - **Hyperprolactinaemia** – stress, micro/macro prolactinoma, other pituitary tumours compressing pituitary stalk, PCOS
  - Drug induced – dopamine antagonists (eg phenothiazines), dopamine depleting agents (eg methyldopa), others (eg oestrogens/OCP)

Purulent

- Breast abscess
- Mastitis
- TB (rare)

> Investigations

Blood tests

- Haematology – FBC, ESR
  - Anaemia (malignancy)
  - Raised WCC (abscess)
  - ESR (tumour, TB)
- Biochemistry
  - U+Es (renal function)
  - CRP (abscess)
  - LFTs (malignancy)
  - Prolactin (hyperprolactinaemia)

Pathology

- Breast secretion
  - Dipstick testing (blood vs other fluid)
  - M,C+S (infection, abscess, TB)
  - Cytology
- FNAC (carcinoma)
- Core (trucut) biopsy

Urine

- β–HCG (pregnancy)

Radiology

- CXR:
  - Metastases
- USS breast (solid vs cystic lump)
- Mammography (carcinoma, duct ectasia)

Further investigations

- X-ray ductogram (papilloma)
- Microdochectomy (intraductal papilloma, intraductal carcinoma)
- CT/MRI Head (prolactinoma of the pituitary gland)

Overdose

The history of the overdose patient requires a collaborative/corroborative history from the patient, relatives, witnesses and ambulance officers.

➤ History of presenting complaint

What is the patient's age and sex?

What was taken?

How much?

How long ago was it taken?

Over what time period?

Where?

Was it accidental, an act of deliberate self harm, or a suicide attempt?

Have you **vomited** since ingestion? How many times? Did you vomit up the tablets?

Did any witnesses see you take it? Who?

Did you take **one drug or more** in combination? Was the overdose staggered? (Serum levels therefore unreliable)

Did you take it alone or **with alcohol**?

Suicidal assessment

How was the patient found? (By chance?)

Did you tell someone before the attempt?

Did you phone the ambulance and, if not, who did?

Was a suicide note found?

Were empty tablet containers found?

What led to the suicide/deliberate self-harm attempt?

What other medications might you have had access to?

Did you want to die? (Was it a cry for help?)

How do you feel about it now? Do you have any regrets? Do you feel silly or disappointed that you failed?

How do you feel about the future? (Socially isolated/loneliness/do they want to try something like this again?)

Associated symptoms

What have the symptoms been since the overdose?

- Sleepiness
- Fits
- Vomiting
- Tinnitus
- Hyperventilation
- Palpitations
- Aspiration

Ask about treatment, if any, already received.

➤ Past medical history

Is there any history of previous suicide attempts/deliberate self-harm? If so, when, how and why?

Is there any history of known psychiatric illness? If so, what treatment were they given?

Is there any history of other significant medical conditions? (Physical illnesses)

➤ *High risk features for paracetamol overdose*

Chronic alcohol abuse

Glutathione depleted state – chronic malnutrition (anorexia nervosa, cystic fibrosis, alcoholism, cachexia, HIV-positive or AIDS) or recent starvation (within 24 hours)

Liver enzyme inducers – carbamazepine, phenobarbital, phenytoin, rifampicin, St John's wort, alcohol, etc

---

➤ Drug history

What are your normal medications?

What other medications do you have access to?

➤ Social history

Do you smoke? How much and for how long?

Do you consume alcohol? How much?

Do you use recreational/illicit drugs?

Occupation (occupational exposures) and access to drugs?

Have you taken time off work? How much?

Manifestations of common overdoses (toxidromes)

Paracetamol	First 24 h: **May have no symptoms**. May get mild N+V, sweating, anorexia 24–36 h: Hepatic necrosis – RUQ pain/tenderness 36–72 h: Recurrence of N+V, jaundice, encephalopathy, renal failure (loin pain, haematuria, proteinuria)
Salicylates	**Unlike paracetamol, many early features:** Restlessness, N+V, dehydration, tinnitus, vertigo, deafness, sweating, warm extremities/flushing, bounding pulses, tremor, hyperventilation
Alcohol	Sedation, confusion, paraesthesia, diplopia, blurred vision, slurred speech, ataxia, nystagmus, respiratory depression, hallucinations, coma
Carbon monoxide	**Drowsiness** is most common. Carbon monoxide levels <20% produce no physiological symptoms, Higher levels may result in (1) headache and nausea (20–30%), (2) confusion (30–40%), (3) coma (40–60%) and (4) death (>60%). The classically described cherry-red skin colour is in fact rare.
Digoxin	**Anorexia (early)**, N+V, diarrhoea, cognitive decline/confusion, palpitations **Visual disturbances**: blurring, flashes, disturbed colour vision (teichopsia/xanthopsia)

Tricyclics	**Anti-ACh effects:** Palpitations (tachycardia), hot dry skin, dry mouth and tongue, dilated pupils, urinary retention, blurred vision, hypotension, hypothermia, flushing, fever **Central effects:** Ataxia, nystagmus, hallucinations, psychosis, seizures (> 5%), drowsiness, respiratory depression, coma
SSRIs	**May have no/mild symptoms.** Drowsiness, agitation, tremor, nystagmus, dizziness, headache, dry mouth, N+V, abdominal pain. Fits (late) **Serotonin syndrome (rare but serious):** hyperpyrexia
Cyanide	Anxiety, agitation, chest tightness, confusion, hyperventilation, SOB, weakness, dizziness, N+V, collapse, convulsions. NB: cyanosis is NOT a feature.
Opiates	Pinpoint pupils, unresponsive, slow respiratory rate, shallow respiration, bradycardia, hypothermia
Benzodiazepines	Drowsiness, ataxia, dysarthria, nystagmus, coma, respiratory depression
β-Blockers	Palpitations (bradycardia), dizziness (hypotension), drowsiness, hallucinations, fits, coma

➤ Investigations

Blood tests

- Haematology – FBC, clotting
  - MCV (alcohol)
  - Clotting/INR (paracetamol)
  - Carboxyhaemoglobin
  - Methaemoglobin
- Biochemistry
  - U+Es (renal function, hypo- and hyperkalaemia)
  - Ca^{2+}, magnesium
  - Glucose
  - LFTs
  - CRP
  - Plasma osmolality (osmolar gap)
  - Paracetamol/salicylate levels (as mixed poisoning is common)

- Digoxin levels
- Lithium levels
- Blood ethanol levels
- Venous bicarbonate
- Cardiac enzymes – troponin I/T
- Arterial blood gases (anion gap)

Urinalysis

- Myoglobinuria due to rhabdomyolysis gives positive stick test for blood

ECG (if hypotension, coexistent heart disease, suspected ingestion of cardiotoxic drugs, or age > 60)

- Angina, non-ST-elevation MI, ST-elevation MI
- Arrhythmias
- Digoxin toxicity
- Changes of hypo- and hyperkalaemia

Radiology

- CXR
  - Aspiration

Further investigations

- Urinary and plasma toxicology
- Specific drug assays as appropriate
- If substance ingested is unknown, save 10 ml serum, 50 ml urine and 50 ml vomitus/first gastric aspirate at 4 °C (in case there is a need for analysis later)

Palpitations

➤ History of presenting complaint

What do you mean by the term palpitations? (Thumping in the chest)

Are you getting palpitations, or an irregular heart beat currently?

Can you tap out the beat?

SOCRATES

Site

Do you feel them in the neck or chest?

Onset

When did they start? (Few minutes ago/years ago)

Have you had them before?

How did it start or finish? (Instantaneously, or over a few minutes)

How frequently do you get them? How long did/do the episode(s) last for? (Seconds/hours)

Is it continuous or intermittent? What is the interval between episodes? (Minutes/days/years)

Character

What was the rate of palpitations? (Fast/normal/slow) Did you take your pulse at the time? What was it?

Was it a regular or an irregular rhythm?

Are you able to tap it out for me on the table please?

Is there any thumping in the chest?

If so, how fast? Is it regular?

Was there a missed beat? (Ectopics)

If so, did the next one feel heavier? ('Pause and thump')

Associated symptoms

- Faintness
- Sweating
- Chest pain
- Breathlessness
- Thumping in the chest or neck
- Loss of consciousness/blackouts/syncope

Was there any post-event polyuria? (Atrial natriuretic peptide production following true arrhythmia)

Are there any other symptoms of cardiac disease?

- Chest pain
- Exertional dyspnoea
- Anxiety
- Orthopnoea
- PND
- Ankle swelling

Are there any symptoms of thyrotoxicosis?

- Tremor
- Sweaty
- Goitre
- Eye signs
- Recent loss of weight

Are there any symptoms of hypothyroidism? (Bradyarrythmias can cause palpitations too)

Are there any symptoms of phaeochromocytoma?

- Flushing
- Tremor
- Headaches
- Sweating

Are there any symptoms of hypoglycaemia?

- Hunger
- Jittery
- Faints
- Palpitations
- Sweaty

- Headache
- Confusion
- Coma

Are there any symptoms of anaemia?

Precipitating factors

What precipitated it? (Strenuous exercise, fright, chest pain?)

Is there any relation to exercise? What effect does exercise have, if any, on the palpitations?

What happens on standing?

Are there any other precipitants – coffee, tea, alcohol, medications? What is your daily intake of caffeine?

When do you get the palpitations – at night when it is quiet?

Do you suffer from anxiety/panic attacks? Do you get any lumps in your throat, tingling in your fingers or around your lips? Do you ever hyperventilate – do you ever feel that you are unable to take a deep breath in, that you can't fill up your lungs fully, or that you are about to suffocate?

Relieving factors

Did anything terminate the palpitations? (Valsalva manoeuvre, medications, or did they end spontaneously?)

Severity

What do you think is wrong?

Are you worried about serious underlying heart disease?

How well are the palpitations tolerated?

Ask about treatment already received, such as aspirin, GTN

What effect do they have on your life?

Cardiovascular risk factors, see Chest pain.

➤ Past medical history

Did you have rheumatic fever as a child?

Is there a history of:

- IHD
- Hypertension
- Angina
- MI
- Collapses
- Pre-syncope
- Previous palpitations
- Cardiac disease or embolic events, eg stroke?

Have you had previous ECG monitoring, 24 hour tapes?

Is there a history of anxiety or depressive disorders?

Is there a history of thyroid disease?

Have you had any pacemakers inserted or implantable loop recorders (eg Reveal devices) inserted?

➤ Drug history

What medications do you take?

Do you take any antiarrhythmics, or drugs with pro-arrhythmic effects, such as digoxin or salbutamol? How often?

Do you take any drugs that could cause electrolyte disturbances? (Such as loop diuretics and hypokalaemia)

Are you on anticoagulants?

Do you drink lots of caffeine? (Tea/coffee/Coke) How much?

➤ Social history

Do you smoke? How much and for how long? When did you stop?

Do you consume much alcohol? (AF/holiday heart syndrome)

Do you use recreational drugs?

How far can you usually walk and what stops you?

How do the symptoms interfere with your life? (Working, sleeping)

➤ Family history

Is there a family history of premature cardiac disease or dysrhythmias?

Differentiating true arrhythmias from sinus tachycardias on the basis of the history

	True arrhythmias	Sinus tachycardias
Speed	Pulse often ≥140	Pulse ≈100
Speed of onset	Instantaneous	Slow – many minutes
Speed of offset	Sudden or slow	Slow
Regularity	Regular or irregular	Regular
Frequency	Often infrequent	Often frequent
Duration	Seconds to minutes	Hours to days
Precipitating factors	Usually none and spontaneous	May or may be none
Anxiety	After palpitations	Before palpitations
SOB	As a result of heart failure	As a result of hyperventilation (acral/circumoral paraesthesia)
Syncope	Possible and ominous	Very rare (vasomotor)
Structural heart disease	More common	Very rare
Valsalva manoeuvre	More frequently useful (supraventricular tachycardias)	Very rarely helpful

Palpitations

➤ Differential diagnosis

Variant of normal

- Increased awareness of normal rhythm
- Often in quiet room (at night)

Cardiovascular

Sinus tachycardias

- **P**hysiological
  - Exercise
  - Stress
  - Pregnancy
- **P**harmacological
  - Adrenaline
  - Thyroxine
  - Atropine
  - Nifedipine
  - Salbutamol
  - Alcohol
  - High caffeine intake
  - Cocaine
- **P**athological
  - Haemorrhage
  - PE
  - CCF
  - Infection/pyrexia
  - Pain
  - Vasovagal syncope
- **P**hysical deconditioning
  - Unfit
  - Depression
  - Chronic fatigue syndromes
  - Anorexia nervosa
  - Weight loss

Cardiac tachyarrhythmias

- Supraventricular tachycardias
  - AF (various causes, eg ischaemic heart disease, thyrotoxicosis, alcohol, mitral valve disease)
  - Atrial flutter
  - Atrial tachycardia
  - Atrioventricular nodal re-entry tachycardia
  - Atrioventricular re-entry tachycardia (Wolff–Parkinson–White syndrome)
  - Pacemaker failure
- Broad-complex tachycardias
  - Monomorphic ventricular tachycardia
  - Polymorphic ventricular tachycardia (torsades de pointes)
- Bradyarrhythmias
  - Intermittent atrioventricular heart block
  - Sinus node disease (sick sinus syndrome) and tachy-brady syndromes
  - Drug-related
    - ➤ Digoxin (bigeminy)
    - ➤ β-Blockers
- Extrasystoles (Ectopic beats)
  - Atrial ectopics
  - Junctional ectopics
  - Ventricular ectopics
- Endocrine
  - Hyperthyroidism
  - Phaeochromocytoma
  - Menopause (due to sudden vasodilatation)
- Metabolic
  - Anaemia
  - Hypoglycaemia
- Psychogenic
  - Anxiety
  - Somatisation

Palpitations

> Investigations

Blood tests
- Haematology – FBC, D-dimers
  - Anaemia (as primary cause or aggravating factor)
  - Raised MCV (alcohol)
  - Raised WCC (infection resulting in AF)
  - D-dimers (PE leading to AF)
- Biochemistry
  - U+Es including Ca^{2+} and magnesium (electrolyte disturbances can precipitate or aggravate arrhythmias)
  - TFTs (sinus tachycardia, AF)
  - Glucose (hypoglycaemia)
  - CRP (infection leading to AF)
  - LFTs (alcohol leading to AF, cardiac cirrhosis)
  - Digoxin levels
  - Cardiac enzymes – troponin I/T (ischaemia)

Microbiology
- Blood cultures (infection triggering arrhythmia)
- Arterial blood gases (PE, pneumonia)

ECG
- Sinus tachycardia
- Arrhythmia (eg supraventricular tachycardia, broad-complex tachycardia, ectopics, etc)
- Ischaemia
- Wolff–Parkinson–White syndrome

24-hour ECG (paroxysmal arrhythmia)

Radiology
- CXR
  - Consolidation
  - CCF
  - Left atrial enlargement (mitral valve disease)
  - Neoplasm

- V/Q scan or CTPA (pulmonary embolus)
- Echocardiography
  - Evidence of structural heart disease
  - Valvular dysfunction
  - Residual LV function
  - Right heart failure (PE)
  - Pulmonary hypertension (PE)
  - Left ventricular hypertrophy (hypertension → AF)

Further investigations

- 24-hour urinary catecholamines (phaeochromocytoma)
- Implantable loop recorders/Cardiomemo devices/Reveal devices (occasional arrhythmias)
- Stress test (ischaemic heart disease)
- Adenosine challenge (arrhythmia subtype analysis)
- Cardiac electrophysiology ± provocation tests (if at particularly high risk)
- Pacemaker check

Pruritus

➤ History of presenting complaint

Site

Is it local or generalised?

Which part of body did it start with?

Are the eyes or anogenital areas involved?

Is there a rash with it?

Is the itch with wheals? (Urticaria)

Onset

Duration of symptoms?

Is it getting better/worse/staying the same?

Associated symptoms

Swollen neck glands, fever, night sweats, weight loss?

Haemoptysis, chronic cough, droopy eyelid, chest pain and weight loss in a smoker? (Bronchial carcinoma)

Is there jaundice? Is there a past history of gallstones? Are the stools pale and the urine dark?

Are there any symptoms of CRF? (Lethargy, anorexia, nocturia, oliguria, polyuria, haematuria, frothy urine, skin fragility, oedema and bone pains)

Are there any features of hyperthyroidism? (Tremor, heat intolerance, palpitations, increased appetite with weight loss, anxiety and diarrhoea)

Are there any features of hypothyroidism? (Cold intolerance, mental slowing, weight gain, constipation and menorrhagia)

Precipitating factors

- Initiation of a drug, alcohol/drug withdrawal
- Hot baths (polycythaemia or aquagenic urticaria)
- Sunlight
- Iron deficiency*
- Skin creams
- Biological washing powders
- Exposure to animals, food (atopy) or irritants (eg fibreglass)

* Therefore ask about any symptoms of blood loss, such as PR bleeding, haematemesis, menorrhagia.

Relieving factors

Are there any relieving factors, such as bath oils?

Severity

Does it affect sleep or work? Is the itching worse during the day or at night?

What do you think is wrong?

Ask about treatment, if any, already received.

➤ Past medical history

Is there any history of previous illnesses or skin conditions?

Are you diabetic?

Is there a past history of anxiety or depression?

➤ Drug history

Do you take any medications?

Prescribed or alternative, ingested or topical?

Are you on the pill (cholestasis), or opiates?

Is there a history of atopy? (Asthma, eczema, hay fever, aspirin sensitivity)

Compliance, side-effect(s) of medication, OTC/herbal remedies, allergies. (What happens?)

➤ Social history

Alcohol intake. Are you dependent on alcohol at all? Is there a history of liver disease?

Do you use recreational drugs? (Opiate-based + withdrawal)

Have you been abroad? (Overseas travel history, tropical illnesses)

Is there anyone in the family with itching, or have you been in contact with anyone with a similar problem of itching?

Have you been in contact with anyone with scabies?

Do you keep animals at home?

What is your occupation? (Occupational exposures such as fibreglass)

How do the symptoms interfere with your life? (Walking, working, sleeping)

➤ Family history

Is there a family history of atopy or skin disorders?

➤ Differential diagnosis

Cutaneous

- Insect/flea bites
- Prickly heat (miliaria rubra)
- Xerosis (dry skin)
  - Age (senile asteatosis)
  - Excessive washing
  - Atopy
  - Drugs
  - Uraemia
- Urticaria
- Eczema
- Contact dermatitis
- Psoriasis
- Infections
  - Scabies
  - Pediculosis and flea bites
  - HSV
  - Herpes zoster
  - Tinea (ringworm)
- Lichen planus
- Pityriasis rosea
- Dermatitis herpetiformis
- Prurigo nodularis (neurodermatitis/lichen simplex chronicus)

Anogenital pruritus

- **All the above causes *plus***
  - Incontinence, diarrhoea, poor hygiene
  - Infection – threadworm, *Candida*, tinea, scabies
  - Haemorrhoids, fissure, fistula, wart
  - Lichen sclerosus
  - Anxiety, tight underwear

Systemic

- Haematological
  - Iron deficiency anaemia
  - Polycythaemia rubra vera
- Cholestatic liver disease
  - Extrahepatic obstruction
  - Intrahepatic obstruction
    - ➤ Primary biliary cirrhosis
    - ➤ Hepatitis
    - ➤ Cirrhosis
    - ➤ Drug-induced cholestasis (OCP)
- Chronic renal failure
- Endocrine disease
  - Thyrotoxicosis
  - Myxoedema
  - Diabetes mellitus
- Malignancy
  - Lymphomas (especially Hodgkin's) and leukaemias
  - Carcinomas
- Drugs
  - Opiates (mast cell degranulation)
  - Alcohol and drug withdrawal
- Tropical infections
  - Filariasis
  - Hookworm
- Pregnancy
- Psychogenic
  - Anxiety neurosis
  - Dermatitis artefacta
  - Psychosis (parasitophobia)

➤ Investigations

Blood tests

- Haematology – FBC, haematinics, blood film, ESR
  - Hb (iron deficiency anaemia, polycythaemia)
  - MCV (microcytic = iron deficiency, normocytic = Hodgkin's)
  - Elevated WCC (leukaemia)
  - Serum iron
  - TIBC (iron deficiency anaemia)
  - Ferritin (iron deficiency)
  - Eosinophils (allergic conditions)
  - Blood film
  - ESR (lymphoma)
- Biochemistry
  - U+Es (renal failure)
  - TFTs (thyroid dysfunction)
  - Glucose (diabetes mellitus)
  - LFTs (cholestasis)

Urinalysis

- Glucose (DM)
- Protein and blood (renal disease)

Skin scrapings

- Mycotic infection, microscopy and culture

Stools

- For blood and parasites

Radiology

- CXR
  - Bilateral hilar lymphadenopathy (Hodgkin's)
  - Bronchial carcinoma
- USS
  - Dilated bile ducts (obstructive jaundice)
  - Size of kidneys, cysts (chronic renal disease)

Pruritus

Further investigations

- Red cell mass (polycythaemia rubra vera)
- Excisional biopsy of lymph node (Hodgkin's disease)
- HIV serology
- Patch testing
- Skin biopsy

Pyrexia of unknown origin and fever

➤ History of presenting complaint

Onset

When did it start?

What were you doing when it started?

Where were you when it started?

Character

Is the fever continuous or cyclical? Is there a pattern? (Malaria, Pel–Ebstein)

Do you feel hot during the fevers?

Associated symptoms

Ask about:

- Pain (abdominal, chest, dysuria, joints, bones and back, headache)
- Breathlessness
- Cough (mild)
- Diarrhoea
- Sore throat
- Jaundice
- Night sweats, pruritus, easy bruising (leukaemias)
- Arthralgia (RA, leukaemia)
- Weight loss, general malaise
- Abdominal masses/lumps or lumps anywhere else? (Abdominal – RCC)

Precipitating factors

Have you been in contact with people/animals with infection/illness?

Have you been in contact with anyone with jaundice?

Have you been in contact with animals, especially farm animals? (Q fever, brucellosis)

Have you had any bites, cuts, abrasions, rashes, calf swelling?

Determine any risk factors for DVT.

Relieving factors

Does paracetamol relieve the fever?

Have you had any trials of aspirin or steroids to control the fever?

What do you think is wrong?

Ask about treatment, if any, already received.

➤ Past medical history

Is there any history of previous illnesses, such as rheumatic fever or IBD?

Has there been any recent surgery, especially abdominal surgery?

Do you have any prosthetic heart valves? (Subacute bacterial endocarditis)

Have you had any transplants? (CMV, lymphoma)

Have you ever had an immunosuppressive illness?

Is there a past history of **SPUR** infections, indicating immunosuppression?

Serious

Protracted

Unusual

Recurrent infections

➤ Drug history

Are you taking any tablets or injections? (Including all non-prescription drugs)

Are you on any immunosuppressants?

Are you taking the pill? (Hepatoma)

Have you had any recent vaccinations? (Immunisation history essential)

Do you have any allergies?

Are you on any non-prescription drugs or drugs of abuse?

Compliance, side-effect(s) of medication, OTC/herbal remedies, allergies. (What happens?)

➤ Social history

Do you use recreational drugs?

Have you ever had tattooing, body piercing or received blood products/transfusions (especially outside the UK)?

A detailed overseas travel history is required, including assessment of tropical illnesses:

- Where did you go?
- When did you go?
- Have you been to any malarial zones in the last year?
- Did you get bitten by any insects/animals, such as ticks, mosquitos, sandflies, dogs?
- Were you ill there?
- Did you take all the malaria prophylaxis and complete the course correctly?
- What did you take?
- Did you put on any insect repellent while away?
- Did you have any vaccinations before travel?
- Where did you stop en route?
- Where did you visit?
- Was it rural or urban? Did you stay in a hotel, campsite, youth hostel?
- What are your leisure activities/pastimes?
- Is there a history of swimming in dirty, fresh water – here or abroad? (Leptospirosis, schistosomiasis).
- What type of food/drink was eaten/drunk abroad? Did you eat seafood (hepatitis A), raw meat, etc? Did you drink the local tap water?

Do you have animals at home or have you been in contact with any animals? Have you been scratched by any cats? (Cat-scratch fever, toxoplasmosis; domestic, farm and wild animals can all be responsible for zoonotic infection)

Are all your immunisations up to date? Have you had any recently?

What is your occupation? (Occupational exposures, exercise capacity, lifestyle limitations due to disease)

Have you had any unprotected sexual intercourse? (HIV/hepatitis risk)

➤ Family history

Is there a family history of malignancy or immune defects?

Is there any IBD in the family?

Has anyone in the family had familial Mediterranean fever?

Has there been any contact with a person with TB or any other infection?

➤ Differential diagnosis

Infectious causes

1. Where is the source of infection?
- Urinary tract
  - **UTI**
  - **Pyelonephritis**
- Chest
  - **Pneumonia**
  - Empyema
- Blood
  - **Septicaemia**
- Brain
  - **Meningitis**
  - Encephalitis
- Heart
  - **Endocarditis**
  - Pericarditis

- Bone and joints
  - **Osteomyelitis**
  - **Septic arthritis**
- GI tract
  - Gastroenteritis
  - Hepatitis
  - **Ascending cholangitis**
- Skin and soft tissue
  - Cellulitis
  - **Surgical wound**
- Abscess (collection) formation
  - Cerebral
  - Chest
  - Abdominal, eg
    - Subphrenic
    - Hepatic
    - Subhepatic
    - Renal and perinephric
    - Paracolic
    - Psoas
    - Appendiceal
    - Diverticular
  - Pelvic
  - Spine
- Intravenous lines (iatrogenic)

2. Which organism is involved?

- In addition to common culprits, also consider:
  - Bacterial – TB, brucellosis, typhoid, leptospirosis, subacute bacterial endocarditis, rheumatic fever
  - Viral – HIV, EBV, viral hepatitis
  - Parasitic – malaria
  - Fungal – histoplasmosis, *Aspergillus*, cryptococcosis

Non-infectious causes

- Neoplasia
  - Lymphomas, leukaemias
  - Other solid tumours – hepatic, renal, lung, pancreatic, disseminated carcinoma
- Connective tissue diseases
  - RA
  - SLE
  - Still's disease
  - Vasculitis, eg PAN, PMR
- Miscellaneous
  - **MI**
  - **DVT/PE**
  - **Anastomotic leak post-op**
  - **Atelectasis**
  - Stroke (hypothalamic dysfunction)
  - **Drug fever/allergy, eg flucloxacillin**
  - **Alcohol withdrawal**
  - **Transfusion reaction**
  - Post-immunisation
  - Inflammatory bowel disease
  - Granulomatous disease (eg sarcoidosis)
  - Hyperthyroidism
  - Familial Mediterranean fever
  - Familial periodic fever
  - Factitious fever
  - Idiopathic

➤ Investigations

Blood tests

- Haematology – FBC, D-dimers, ESR, blood film
  - Anaemia (malignancy, anaemia of chronic disease)
  - Raised WCC (infection, inflammation, leukaemia)
  - Thrombocytopenia (leukaemia)
  - D-dimers (DVT/PE)

- ESR (malignancy, connective tissue disease, TB)
- Blood films (thick and thin) (blood dyscrasias, malaria)
- Serum immuno-electrophoresis (myeloma)
- Biochemistry
  - U+Es (connective tissue disease with renal involvement)
  - Glucose (diabetes increases risk of infection)
  - CRP (infection)
  - LFTs (biliary tract or liver disease)
  - Tumour markers (PSA, CA 19-9, CA 125, CEA)
- Immunology
  - Rheumatoid factor (RA)
  - Autoimmune profile (connective tissue disease)

Microbiology

- Three blood cultures at different sites and different times (infective endocarditis, sepsis)
- Viral antibodies (hepatitis B/C, EBV (Paul–Bunnell), CMV, HIV)
- Sputum culture (AAFBs, M,C+S)
- Mantoux test (TB)
- Stool culture and microscopy (M,C+S, ova, cysts and parasites)
- Serology (Q fever, brucellosis, leptospirosis, syphilis)
- Three consecutive early-morning MSUs (TB)

Urinalysis

- M,C+S
- Glucose (DM)
- Blood (endocarditis, RCC, blood dyscrasias)
- Pus cells (infection)
- Proteinuria (suggests renal disease)
- Granular or red cell casts (renal inflammation, eg connective tissue disorder)

ECG

- Cardiac disease

Radiology

- CXR
  - TB
  - Occult infection/atypical pneumonia
  - Pneumonitis (HIV, *Pneumocystis carinii* pneumonia)
  - Malignancy (eg lung, lymphoma)
  - Hilar enlargement (sarcoidosis, TB, lymphoma)

Further investigations

- Antistreptolysin O titre (rheumatic fever)
- Bone marrow aspirate/trephine biopsy (leukaemia, myeloma)
- Lumbar puncture (meningitis, SAH, Guillain–Barré syndrome)
- Transthoracic/transoesophageal echocardiography (endocarditis)
- USS abdomen (occult intra-abdominal collection, malignancy)
- Gallium scan/labelled WCC scan (localised infection)
- MRI pituitary/hypothalamus (hypothalamic dysfunction from invading pituitary tumour)
- Liver biopsy (hepatitis)
- Renal biopsy (glomerular disease, malignancy)
- Muscle biopsy (myositis)
- Temporal artery biopsy (giant cell arteritis)
- CT chest/abdomen (occult infection, malignancy)
- Exploratory laparotomy (intra-abdominal sepsis)

Rashes

➤ History of presenting complaint

Site

Where is it?

Is it localised or generalised?

Onset

When was the rash first noticed?

How long have you had it?

Is this the first time it has occurred? When does it occur? (Weekdays, weekends, away from home/on holiday, at home, in bed?)

Is there any pattern to where and when it occurs? (The timing of change is important, especially for moles)

Character

Determine the exact pattern of the rash – is it grouped, scattered, linear, annular, etc? Are there single or multiple lesions?

What is the shape, size and colour of the lesion?

Is it flat or raised? Does the lesion seem to be fluid-filled?

What is the rate of progression of the rash? Is it getting better, worse or remaining static?

What is the mode of spread with time? (For example annular or irregular spread) Does the rash move around? Is it fluctuating or persistent? How long does the rash or lesion last for?

Is the rash symmetrical? (Implies endogenous cause)

Is the rash asymmetrical? (Implies exogenous cause)

Are the borders of the lesions well-defined or ill-defined?

Are the flexures/skin creases involved?

Is the hair, or are the nails or mucous membranes (mouth, eyes, genitalia) affected? (Mouth ulcers may been seen in SLE or gluten enteropathy)

How does it bother you?

Associated symptoms

Is it itchy? Is there any scaling? Are you repeatedly rubbing it? (Itch–scratch–itch cycle)

Is there any pain, tenderness or soreness? (Inflammation, tumours)

What are the surface characteristics – is there any weeping, scaling, crusting or blistering?

Does it smell?

Is the skin hotter or colder than usual?

Are there any lumps? (Where is the lump? Is it itchy? Has it bled? Has its shape/size/colour changed? Are there any other lumps?)

Is there a colour change? What is the colour change? (Increased pigmentation, jaundice, pallor) Who noticed it? How long ago did they notice it? Do you have any old photos?

Does the redness disappear (blanch) with light pressure? That is, is it erythema (disappears) or purpura (persists)?

Do you have any joint pain? (Psoriatic arthropathy, vasculitis)

Do you have any urinary tract symptoms, such as haematuria? (Vasculitis)

Are there any associated systemic features, such as weight loss, arthralgia or fever?

Precipitating factors

Were there any precipitants, such as medication, diet, sunlight? (Herpes/SLE/vitiligo) Potential allergens, physical/chemical agents? (At home or at work) Cold, heat, stress, infections? (Such as a sore throat prior to guttate psoriasis)

Does anything happen at sites of trauma, such as scratches or scars? (Koebner phenomenon)

Do you remember being bitten by an insect?

Has anyone else in the family, or at work, been affected by a similar rash? (This includes all contacts – family, friends and colleagues)

Have you had recent sun exposure – do you sit in sun? Do you burn easily? Do you use a high-factor suncream? Do you use sunbeds? Do you travel a lot? Do you wear a sunhat when abroad?

What do you think is wrong?

Ask about treatment, if any, already received, such as steroids, antihistamines, topical creams? How was the treatment used?

➤ Past medical history

Is there any history of previous rashes, such as psoriasis?

Is there a history of atopic tendencies? (Asthma, eczema, rhinitis, aspirin sensitivity)

Do you have any allergies to nuts and food?

Do you have allergies to washing powders or soap?

Did you have any skin problems in childhood?

Is there a history of other medical conditions, such as SLE, coeliac disease, myositis, renal transplantation, psoriatic arthropathy?

Is there a history of varicose veins/deep vein thrombosis? (Venous eczema)

➤ Drug history

As a general rule, any drug can cause any skin reaction.

Are you taking any tablets or injections, prescribed and alternative, ingested and topical?

Are you taking lithium, β-blockers or antimalarials? (May precipitate psoriasis)

What previous treatments have you taken for the skin disorder?

Are you using immunosuppressants? (Skin tumours)

Do you have any allergies to medication? If so, what was the reaction? Do you know of any possible allergens?

Have you undergone any patch testing or IgE responses?

Compliance, side-effect(s) of medication, OTC/herbal remedies, allergies. (What happens?)

➤ Social history

Do you consume alcohol?

Do you use recreational drugs?

Have you been abroad recently? (Overseas travel history, tropical illnesses) Have you ever lived in a hot/sunny country? Where did you grow up as a child? Did you get sunburnt a lot as a child?

Do you keep any animals at home or pets? Have you been in contact with any farm animals?

What is your occupation? (Occupational exposures) Do you work outdoors?

Have you been exposed to sunlight, potential allergens, skin parasites?

Have you changed washing products, pets, etc?

Have you been exposed to infectious conditions such as chickenpox? Does anyone you know (family or friends) have (or did they have) a similar rash?

What are your hobbies? Do you play contact sports? (Where infectious causes are more likely, such as herpes gladiatorum, impetigo, tinea)

➤ Family history

Is there a family history of skin disorders/atopy? Are there any others in the family affected by this?

Is there a family history of eczema or psoriasis?

Is there a family history of other skin disorders?

➤ Differential diagnosis

Remember any drug can cause any skin reaction.

Erythrosquamous eruptions

- Infectious
  - Bacterial
    - ➤ **Cellulitis**
    - ➤ Erysipelas
    - ➤ **Impetigo**
    - ➤ Staphylococcal scalded skin syndrome
    - ➤ Secondary syphilis
    - ➤ Lyme (erythema chronicum migrans)
  - Viral
    - ➤ Measles
    - ➤ Rubella
    - ➤ Parvovirus B19
    - ➤ Molluscum contagiosum
    - ➤ HPV warts
  - Fungal
    - ➤ **Ringworm** (tinea/dermatophyte infections)
    - ➤ *Candida*
  - Parasitic
    - ➤ **Scabies**
    - ➤ Pediculosis
- Eczema/dermatitis
  - Exogenous dermatitis
    - ➤ **Primary irritant contact dermatitis**
    - ➤ **Allergic contact dermatitis**
  - Endogenous dermatitis
    - ➤ **Atopic**
    - ➤ **Seborrhoeic**
    - ➤ Discoid
    - ➤ Asteatotic
    - ➤ Pompholyx
    - ➤ Venous/varicose

Psoriasis

- **Classical plaque** (nummular)
- **Guttate**
- Erythrodermic
- Generalised acute pustular
- Chronic palmo-plantar pustulosis
- Arthropathic
- Urticaria
- Erythroderma
- Erythema nodosum
- Pityriasis rosea
- Lichen planus
- **Drug reaction** (eg toxic epidermal necrolysis, fixed drug reaction)
- Tumours:
  - Solar (actinic) keratosis
  - Bowen's disease
  - Paget's disease
  - Superficial basal cell carcinoma
  - Mycosis fungoides
- Psychogenic (dermatitis artefacta)

Blistering skin diorders

- **Insect bites**
- Traumatic/burns
- Infectious:
  - Viral
    - HSV
    - **Varicella zoster**
    - Chickenpox
  - Bacterial
    - Bullous impetigo
  - Parasitic
    - Scabies
- Eczema herpeticum
- Bullous eczema and pompholyx
- Erythema multiforme
- Dermatitis herpetiformis

- Bullous Pemphigoi**D** (**D**eeper)
- Pemphigu**S** (**S**uperficial)
- Porphyria cutanea tarda
- Drug reaction

Hypopigmentation
- Post-inflammatory
- **Vitiligo**
- **Pityriasis versicolor**
- Leprosy

Photodistributed
- **Sunburn**
- **Drug reaction** (eg amiodarone, tetracyclines)
- **SLE**
- Dermatomyositis
- Porphyria cutanea tarda
- Pellagra
- Phototoxicity (eg phytophotodermatitis)
- Photosensitive eczema/chronic actinic dermatitis
- Polymorphic light eruption
- **Carcinomas**

Tumours
- An external rash may represent the presence of an **internal** malignancy
- Important skin tumours never to miss include:
    - **Squamous cell carcinoma**
    - **Basal cell carcinoma** (rodent ulcer)
    - **Malignant melanoma**

> Investigations

Blood tests

- Haematology – FBC, ESR
  - Anaemia (SLE and other connective tissue disorders)
  - Raised WCC (infection)
  - Leucopenia (SLE)
  - ESR (inflammation, infection, malignancy, connective tissue disorder)
- Biochemistry
  - U+Es (renal dysfunction in drug reactions, connective tissue disorders, vasculitides)
  - Glucose (DM → candidiasis and other rashes)
  - CRP (infection)
  - LFTs (if palmar erythema)
  - TFTs (if palmar erythema, pre-tibial myxoedema)
  - Lipids (xanthomata)
- Virology
  - HIV, measles, rubella, parvovirus, herpes, varicella

Microbiology

- Blood cultures (infective)
- Syphilis serology (VDRL)
- Lyme serology
- Antistreptolysin O titres (erythema nodosum)
- Skin scrapings (M,C+S for fungal and bacterial isolation, fluorescence under Wood's light, cytology for carcinoma)
- Swab pus/crusting/exudates/vesicular fluid

Histology

- Skin biopsy (punch biopsy or incision/excision biopsy)

Immunology

- Autoimmune profile – ANA, anti-dsDNA, antinucleosome, anti-Ro and anti-La antibodies, rheumatoid factor, serum complement, anticardiolipin antibodies and raised immunoglubulins (SLE)
- Complement, C1 esterase inhibitor (angioneurotic oedema/ urticaria)

Urinalysis

- Proteinuria (inflammatory or vasculitic lesions)
- Glucose (DM)

Radiology

- CXR (TB, sarcoidosis and erythema nodosum)

Further investigations

- Skin allergy testing
- Patch testing (delayed hypersensitivity response)
- Prick/scratch testing (immediate hypersensitivity response)

Red eye

> ## History of presenting complaint

Site

Is it **unilateral** or **bilateral**?

Onset

How long has the eye been red?

Was the onset **sudden** or **gradual**?

Associated symptoms

Is there discomfort or irritation?

Is it **painful**?

Is it worse with eye movement? (Scleritis)

Is there a headache with it?

Is the **vision impaired** at all? (Visual acuity)

Is the eye 'sticky'?

Is there any exudate? (Presence, amount, colour)

Is the eye watering? (Cluster headaches, iritis, keratitis)

Is the dark of the eye (pupil) or eyelid(s) affected?

Is the eye dry or gritty?

Are there any systemic features, eg fever, malaise, vomiting, arthralgia, rashes, headache or facial pain?

Is there any photophobia? (Iritis, keratitis, glaucoma)

Is there any urethral discharge/arthralgia? (Reiter's syndrome)

Precipitating factors

Is there a history of foreign body insertion or trauma?

Is there any eye itching or seasonal variation?

Does anyone in the family have eye symptoms? (For example, transmission of viral conjunctivitis from sharing towels)

What do you think is wrong?

Ask about treatment, if any, already received.

➤ Past medical history

Is there any previous history of eye problems?

Is there a history of hay fever? (Atopy)

Have you had previous herpes infection on the face?

Do you wear contact lenses?

Is there a history of RA/SLE/IBD/psoriasis/AS/sarcoid/thyroid eye disease?

Have you had recent cataract surgery?

Is there any previous history of known illnesses, eg sarcoid, immunosuppression?

➤ Drug history

Do you take any medications, such as eye drops (eg for glaucoma)?

Do you take any eye drops that you may be allergic to, or which may cause disease (preservatives)?

Compliance, side-effect(s) of medication, OTC/herbal remedies, allergies. (What happens?)

➤ Social history

Sexual history. (Reiter's syndrome)

➤ Family history

Is there a family history of glaucoma?

> Differential diagnosis

Unilateral

- Painless
  - Episcleritis
  - Subconjunctival/conjunctival haemorrhage
  - Chalazion
- Painful
  - **Scleritis** (→ scleromalacia perforans in RA)
  - Corneal abrasion/erosion/trauma
  - Trichiasis
  - **Foreign body**
  - **Iritis (anterior uveitis)**
  - **Periorbital cellulitis**
  - Acute keratitis/corneal ulcer/dendritic ulcer
  - **Acute angle-closure glaucoma**
  - Hordeolum and styes
  - Cluster headache (migrainous neuralgia)

Bilateral

- Painless
  - Infectious/allergic conjunctivitis
  - Ectropion/entropion
  - Keratoconjunctivitis sicca
  - Thyroid eye disease (chemosis)
- Painful
  - Blepharitis

Red eye

➤ Investigations

Blood tests

- Haematology – FBC, ESR
  - Raised WCC (inflammation)
  - ESR (inflammation, eg uveitis)
- Biochemistry
  - TFTs (thyroid eye disease)
  - Glucose (diabetes mellitus)
  - CRP (infection)
- Immunology
  - Rheumatoid factor (RA)
  - HLA-B27 typing
  - Autoimmune profile

Microbiology

- Eye swabs (M,C+S)

Other

- Slit lamp examination
- Tonometry (glaucoma)
- Corneal scrapings

Further investigations

- CXR, serum Ca^{2+}, serum ACE (sarcoidosis → uveitis)
- Syphilis (VDRL) serology (uveitis)

Scrotal pain and swellings

➤ History of presenting complaint

NB How old are you? (assume torsion until proven otherwise in the young)

Site

What exactly have you noticed? (lump, feeling of heaviness down below, pain, dragging ache etc?).

Onset

When did you first notice it?

Was the onset sudden or gradual?

How long have you had it?

How did you notice the swelling?

Has it got bigger or worse over time, stayed the same or got better?

How many hours ago did the pain start? (torsion)

What were you doing at the time that the pain or swelling started (vigorous exercise or cycling for example)? Was it first noticed by yourself?

Character

Where exactly is the pain or swelling?

Right or left hand side?

Where do you feel it originates from – within the testicle itself or in a different part of the scrotum? Can you feel the lump separately from the testicle? What is the consistency, size, shape? Is it smooth?

Radiation

Does the pain radiate to the groin or abdomen? (as in testicular torsion or ureteric colic)

Associated symptoms

Have you had any masses associated with the testicle prior to the onset of the pain? (tumours)

Have you noticed any other lumps, eg in the groin/abdomen/neck (LNs)?

Is the lump tender/painful, or painless?

Do you have any abdominal pain?

Have you had any nausea and vomiting?

Have you had any recent facial pain/swellings/pain upon eating? (parotitis in mumps orchitis)

Does the lump or pain change with position in any way – lying, sitting etc? (varicocele, hernia). Can you make the lump disappear at all?

Does elevation of the testicle affect the pain in any way? (**Prehn's sign** – in torsion, pain is exacerbated by lifting up the testis, in epididymitis the pain is relieved by lifting the testis).

Is the testis retracted, in a different position to normal, or in its normal position? (torsion)

Have you noticed any skin/surface changes such as redness, heat or itching?

Are there any **urinary symptoms** such as dysuria, frequency, urgency, urge incontinence, urinary retention?

Is there any penile discharge, penile ulcers/warts, haematuria, haematospermia?

Have you come into contact with anyone with TB?

Are there any systemic features –

- fever
- malaise/lethargy
- anorexia
- weight loss
- swollen glands
- back pain (enlarged para-aortic LNs, torsion)
- cough
- haemoptysis
- SOB (lung metastases, TB)

- sweats
- gynaecomastia (testicular tumours)

Are there any features of **bowel obstruction** (strangulated hernia) –

- vomiting
- distension
- colicky abdominal pain
- absolute constipation (failure to pass flatus or faeces)

Precipitating factors

Is there a history of trauma, infections?

What do you think is wrong?

Ask about treatment, if any, already received?

➤ Past medical history

Have you ever had any problems with either or both testes?

Is there a history of maldescended testes (one or both sides? Which side?), or other congenital abnormalities such as hydroceles?

Have you had mumps before?

Have you had previous testicular carcinoma?

Is there a history of torsion in the contralateral testis?

Is there a history of sexually transmitted diseases?

Have you ever had a hernia?

➤ Drug history

Have you been on any recent antibiotics?

➤ Social history

Do you smoke?

Do you consume much alcohol?

Do you use recreational drugs?

> Sexual history

Have you had/do you have a regular sexual partner? Have you had any other sexual partners? How is your partner? Have you had recent unprotected sex? (Epididymitis)

Are you currently trying for a baby? Do you have any children? (varicoceles and orchitis are associated with infertility)

Overseas travel history and sexual history abroad.

How do the symptoms interfere with your life (sex, walking, working, sleeping)?

> Family history

Is there a FHx of testicular cancer?

> Differential diagnosis

Scrotal pain

- **Testicular torsion**
- **Epididymo-orchitis**
  - Bacterial: Coliforms, UTI, STIs (*Chlamydia*), syphilis
  - Viral: Mumps, glandular fever
- **Tumours**
- **Trauma (haematocele)**
- **Torsion of the appendix testis (hydatid of Morgagni)**
- **Incarcerated/strangulated inguino-scrotal hernia**
- Epididymal cyst
- Varicocele
- Hydrocele
- Referred pain
  - **Ureteric colic**
- Granulomatous conditions:
  - TB
  - Sarcoid
- Vasculitis:
  - Polyarteritis nodosa

- Henoch-Schönlein purpura
- Fournier's gangrene

Scrotal Swellings

1. Where you can get above the swelling and it is **confined** to the testis:
- **Testicular torsion**
- **Hydrocele (vaginal)**
- **Epididymo-orchitis**
- Haematocele
- **Tumour**
- Syphilitic gumma, TB

2. Where you can get above the swelling but it remains **separate** from the testis:
- Sebaceous cyst
- **Epididymal cyst**
- **Epididymitis**
- **Varicocele**
- Spermatocele
- Encysted hydrocele of the cord

3. Where you **cannot** get above the swelling:
- **Indirect inguinal hernia**
- Infantile hydrocele

➤ Investigations

Blood tests

- Haematology: FBC, ESR
  - anaemia (anaemia of chronic disease)
  - raised WCC (infection)
  - ESR (inflammation, infection, carcinoma, PAN)
- Biochemistry:
  - U+Es (renal function, ascites/cardiac failure → swelling)
  - LFTs (metastases)
  - Ca^{2+} (metastases and sarcoid)
  - Serum ACE (sarcoid)

- Tumour markers:
  - Alpha fetoprotein (teratoma)
  - β –HCG (seminoma)
  - LDH

Urine dipstick

- UTI associated with epididymo-orchitis (blood, protein, leukocytes, nitrites)
- Blood (referred pain from ureteric calculus)

Microbiology

- Urine culture: UTI associated with epididymo-orchitis
- Three consecutive early morning MSUs (TB)
- Urethral swabs for M,C&S (*Gonococcus*, *Chlamydia*)
- Syphilis serology (VDRL)
- Mumps, EBV serology (Monospot/Paul-Bunnell test)

Radiology

- Scrotal USS ± FNAC
  - Solid vs cystic swellings
  - Arising from the body of the testis or not
  - Pathology (solid tumour, hydrocele, haematocele, epididymal cyst, varicocele)
- Abdominal X-ray (referred pain from ureteric stone)
- Abdominal USS (Left RCC → left varicocele)
- Chest X-ray (cannonball metastases, sarcoid, TB)
- CT/MRI thorax, abdomen, pelvis (metastases, staging)

Further investigations

- Angiography: Microaneurysms in PAN
- Laser Doppler/technetium scan: Torsion versus epididymo-orchitis. Absent testicular blood flow in testicular torsion (rarely time for investigation – testis dies within 6 hrs of onset of pain!)
- Laparoscopy (retroperitoneoscopy): to assess abdominal lymph nodes
- Exploratory surgery: definitive and mandatory for testicular torsion

Shortness of breath

➤ History of presenting complaint

Onset

How long have you been breathless for?

How did it start – gradually or slowly? (Determine pattern)

Is it getting better/worse/staying the same?

Character

Is there any diurnal variation?

Is it worse during the day or at night?

Weekdays or weekends? What about during holidays?

Does it come and go (fluctuating), or is it constant? Is it progressive?

Associated symptoms

General symptoms

- Fever
- Night sweats
- Anorexia
- Weight loss
- Lethargy
- Malaise
- Confusion
- Myalgias
- Rigors
- Fatigue
- Swollen glands

Do you have any chest pain, chest tightness or pain on deep inspiration? What came first, the chest pain or breathlessness?

Do you have a cough? (Duration) Is it present at any particular time of day?

Do you wheeze (and when)? Is there any associated flushing? (Carcinoid syndrome)

Do you bring up any sputum? (Quantity, colour, smell/taste, frothiness)

Do you have haemoptysis? (Distinguish from haematemesis and nasopharyngeal bleeding)

Do you have stridor or noisy breathing? (Inspiratory or expiratory)

Is it mainly a problem breathing in? (Foreign body) Or when you try to breathe out? (Asthma/COPD)

Is there a history of any recent chest infections/pneumonias/viral illnesses?

Do you have a droopy eyelid/absence of sweating on one side of face, wasting of hand muscles, hoarsness of your voice, thirstiness? (Ca^{2+}) Do you think you have jaundice, do you have abdominal tenderness, bone pain, headaches? (Metastatic lung cancer)

Are there any symptoms of OSA? (Morning headaches, daytime sleepiness, snoring)

Cardiovascular

- Palpitations
- Ankle swelling
- Syncope

Sputum (quantity, colour, smell/taste, frothiness)

Orthopnoea and PND – Do you have problems with your breathing at night? How many pillows do you sleep with? What happens if you lie flat?

Gastrointestinal

- Has there been any diarrhoea? (Carcinoid)
- Is there a history of possible foreign body or vomitus aspiration? Has there been a period of LOC? (Aspiration pneumonia)

Are there any skin lesions, or is there joint or eye involvement? (Sarcoid, fibrosis, connective tissue diseases, etc)

Is there associated atopy – eczema, allergic rhinitis/hay fever, nasal polyps, asthma, aspirin sensitivity?

Precipitating factors

Do you get short of breath at work or on holiday? (Potential allergen at work?)

Is there any seasonal variation? Is it worse in winter? (COPD) Or in summer? (Pollen)

What were you doing when it started? (Lying down, running, walking, lifting, etc)

What brings it on ('trigger factors')?

- Exercise (asthma)
- Cold air
- Allergens
- Feathery or furry animals
- Pollen, dust
- Infections
- Chemicals
- Irritants
- Smoky environments
- Lying down

Do you suffer from anxiety/panic attacks? Do you get any lumps in your throat, tingling in your fingers or around your lips? Do you ever hyperventilate? Do you ever feel that you are unable to take a deep breath in, that you cannot fill up your lungs fully, or that you are about to suffocate?

Relieving factors

Posture?

Medication (salbutamol, oxygen)?

Does your inhaler help at this time? What is your technique like?

Severity

Try to engage in the severity by asking about nocturnal symptoms, symptoms with exercise – How often do you use your inhaler? How many prescriptions do you go through? Have you had any days/time off work or school?

In the last week or month have you had difficulty sleeping because of your symptoms? Has your breathlessness interfered with your usual daily activities? (Such as housework, work, school)

Do you have a peak flow meter at home? If so, what are your (normal) readings like?

What is the main symptom? Which is the worst for you?

What is your exercise tolerance?

How far can you walk on the flat, or in terms of the number of flights of stairs you are able to climb? What stops you?

What does the breathlessness stop you doing?

> ### ➤ *Risk factors for DVT/PE*
>
> (*most significant)
>
> **Intrinsic** (patient-based) (non-modifiable):
> Age*, hereditary thrombophilic disorders, antiphospholipid syndrome, past history DVTs/PEs*, chronic venous insufficiency, morbid obesity*, CCF, malignancy*, pregnancy and post-partum, polycythaemia, nephrotic syndrome, splenectomy
>
> **Extrinsic** (environmental) (modifiable):
> Recent operations/surgery, trauma and fractures, immobility*, long-haul flights, OCP/HRT, TEDs/heparin prophylaxis not being given in hospital, smoking, dehydration
>
> Do you have swollen and/or painful calves? (Suggestive of a DVT)

Cardiovascular risk factors, see Chest pain.

What do you think is wrong? What are your concerns? (Losing his/her job because of ill health?)

Ask about treatment, if any, already received.

➤ Past medical history

Have you ever been hospitalised?

Are there any systemic conditions – RA, AS, TB, systemic sclerosis, radiation exposure?

Have you had any exposure to TB?

Have you ever had an abnormal chest X-ray?

Are you waiting for any operations at the moment and would your breathing affect the operation going ahead in any way?

Have there been any previous episodes like this one? Have you had a previous pneumothorax, or collapsed lung?

Have you ever had a DVT or PE?

Have you ever needed ventilation? Why?

Is there a history of cardiovascular or respiratory diseases, especially heart failure, asthma, COPD, PEs?

Are there any potential causes of acidosis – DKA, renal failure?

Do you have any allergies? (Which could trigger anaphylaxis) Have you had an anaphylactic reaction in the past? Is there a history of foreign body aspiration?

Do you smoke? Have you ever smoked? If so, how many?

Did you have any lung diseases in childhood, such as recurrent chest infections or TB?

Have you had any previous ECG monitoring or 24-hour tape results?

Is your immune system depressed? (Immunosuppression)

Have you had a BCG vaccination/Mantoux test or a history of diagnosed TB?

Have you ever had treatment for TB? If so, what agents were given and what was the duration of treatment? What was compliance like and **was TB therapy directly observed**?

➤ Drug history

What treatments have you taken for it?

Do any drugs make the breathlessness worse? (NSAIDs, β-blockers, ACE inhibitors)

Is there exposure to drugs with respiratory side-effects? (Amiodarone and pulmonary fibrosis, for example)

Do you use home oxygen? What percentage oxygen, or how many litres a minute do you use? Do you use oxygen cylinders, or do you have a concentrator? For how many hours a day do you use the oxygen? Do you use it at night? Do you take it out of the house with you?

Do you use home nebulisers or inhalers ('preventers' and/or 'relievers') of any sort?

Do you know how to use your inhalers correctly? Have you ever been taught how to use them properly?

Do you use a spacer device with your inhalers?

Is there a history of worsening breathlessness after use of aspirin/NSAIDs, β-blockers (including glaucoma drops)?

Side-effect(s) of medications (steroid inhalers → hoarse voice and *Candida*, β$_2$ agonists → palpitations and tremor). Compliance, OTC/herbal remedies, allergies (pets, medications, dust mites). (What happens?)

➤ Social history

Do you smoke? How much and for how long? When did you stop? (Ask if they have tried to stop or congratulate them for stopping) Ask about previous, current and passive smoking exposure (at home and at work).

Do you drink alcohol?

Do you use recreational drugs?

Have you been overseas recently (TB, *Legionella*, etc), or have you had any tropical illnesses?

Do you have any animals at home? Birds? Parrots? Budgerigars?

What are your hobbies? (A hobby may be implicated in respiratory illness, or a respiratory condition may affect the continuation of such a hobby in the future, eg pigeon racing and EAA, deep-sea diving and pneumothorax, etc)

What is your occupation (and its exposures), and have you had any previous occupations? What tasks were performed at work and what materials were used?

Do the symptoms show a direct relationship to exposure to the work environment?

What is your exercise capacity, and what are your lifestyle limitations due to disease? Has the breathlessness interfered with any activities?

Has there been any deterioration in breathlessness at work/home? Do you get relief on holidays/at weekends, etc? Is your workplace/home near any building sites? (Asbestos, *Aspergillus* spores, etc)

Have you taken any days off work or school due to breathlessness? Is your sleep disturbed?

Have there been any occupational exposures, eg **asbestos**, pneumoconiosis, coal dust, hay, cotton, hobbies and pigeons?

Have you ever been exposed to asbestos, dust or other toxins?

What can't you do physically that you would like to do?

What is your usual exercise tolerance? How far can you usually walk and what stops you?

Are you able to get out of the house? Can you climb the stairs? Where is your bed/bathroom, etc? Who does the shopping, washing, cooking?

How do the symptoms interfere with your life? (Walking, working, sleeping)

➤ Family history

Is there a family history of thrombophilia?

Are there any hereditary lung conditions? (Cystic fibrosis, Kartagener's syndrome, α_1-antitrypsin deficiency, etc)

Is there a personal or family history of asthma or atopy? (Eczema, allergic rhinitis/hay fever, asthma, aspirin sensitivity)

Is there a family history of TB? (Environmental rather than a genetic link)

Differentiating asthma from COPD on the basis of the history

COPD	Asthma
Onset in mid-life (> 35 years old)	Onset early in life (< 35 years old)
Symptoms slowly progressive	Symptoms vary from day to day
Long smoking history	Symptoms often at night/early morning
Chronic productive cough	May have associated allergic disease
Dyspnoea persistent and progressive	May have positive family history
Largely *irreversible* airflow limitation	Largely *reversible* airflow limitation

> Differential diagnosis

Sudden (seconds–minutes)

- Inhaled foreign body
- Aspiration
- Anaphylaxis
- Chest trauma (haemothorax)
- Myocardial infarction
- Dissecting aneurysm
- Pulmonary oedema
- Cardiac arrhythmia
- Pneumothorax
- Acute asthma attack
- Pulmonary embolus
- Panic attack

Acute (hours–days)

- Asthma
- Respiratory tract infection (bacterial, viral, fungal, TB)
- Acute exacerbation of COPD
- Left ventricular failure (pulmonary oedema)
  - LV dysfunction
  - Valvular dysfunction (infective endocarditis)
  - Septal rupture post-MI

- Lung carcinoma
  - Primary
  - Metastatic (especially breast, kidney, sarcoma, melanoma)
- Pleural effusion
- Lobar collapse
- Respiratory muscle weakness (Guillain–Barré)
- Metabolic acidosis (eg DKA, blood loss)

Chronic (months–years)

- COPD
- Bronchiectasis
- Lung carcinoma
  - Primary
  - Metastatic (especially breast, kidney, sarcoma, melanoma)
- Diffuse parenchymal lung disease
  - Pulmonary fibrosis
    - Cryptogenic
    - Connective tissue disease
    - Drugs
    - Environmental
    - Occupational
  - Extrinsic allergic alveolitis
- Anaemia
- Cardiac disease
  - CCF
  - Arrhythmia
  - Valvular heart disease
- Chest wall deformities and obesity
- Eosinophilic pneumonia
- Sarcoidosis
- Main airway obstruction
- Physical deconditioning (from any illness)
- Neuromuscular disorders
  - Muscular dystrophy
  - Motor neurone disease

- Pulmonary hypertension
  - Primary
  - Secondary
    - Interstitial lung disease
    - Recurrent pulmonary thromboembolic disease
    - COPD

Investigations

Blood tests

- Haematology – FBC, D-dimers, ESR
  - Anaemia as primary cause or exacerbating factor (eg bleeding)
  - Raised WCC (pneumonia)
  - Differential WCC (infection, eosinophilia)
  - D-dimers (PE)
  - ESR (carcinoma, infection, inflammation)
- Biochemistry
  - U+Es (SIADH, renal dysfunction → CCF)
  - Ca^{2+} (sarcoidosis)
  - Glucose (DKA, increased risk of LRTI in diabetes)
  - CRP (infection)
  - Serum ACE (sarcoid)
  - LFTs (cardiac cirrhosis, atypical pneumonia, disseminated carcinoma)
  - Cardiac enzymes – troponin I/T (silent MI)
- Immunology
  - Autoimmune screen and autoantibodies (SLE, fibrosing alveolitis, RA, scleroderma, etc)

Arterial blood gases

- Type 1 vs type 2 respiratory failure
- Metabolic acidosis
- Alveolar–arterial oxygen concentration gradient (PE)

Microbiology

- Blood cultures (pneumonia, TB, sepsis)
- Paired serology (atypical infections)
- Sputum culture (including AAFBs)
- *Aspergillus* precipitins
- Serum precipitins (EAA)
- Mantoux/Heaf test (TB)

ECG

- MI
- Arrhythmia
- PE

Urinalysis

- Glucose, ketones (DKA)
- Urinary antigen detection available for *Pneumococcus*, *Legionella* or *Chlamydia*

Peak flow (best of three)

Pulmonary function tests

- Spirometry (obstructive vs restrictive defect)
- Reversibility (COPD vs asthma)
- Flow-volume loops
- Transfer factor

Radiology

- CXR
  - Pulmonary oedema
  - Pneumonia/aspiration pneumonitis
  - TB
  - COPD
  - Pneumothorax
  - Neoplasm (primary or secondaries)
  - Pulmonary fibrosis
  - Pleural effusion

- Lobar collapse
- Sarcoidosis
- (High-resolution) CT thorax
  - Interstitial lung disease/fibrosis
  - Bronchiectasis
  - Staging of neoplasm
  - V/Q scan or CTPA (pulmonary embolus)
- Echocardiography
  - Valvular dysfunction
  - Cardiac failure/LV dysfunction
  - Pulmonary hypertension/right heart failure (PE, interstitial lung disease, COPD, primary pulmonary hypertension)

Further investigations

- Fibreoptic bronchoscopy – diagnostic and therapeutic
  - Cytology – bronchial brushings, washings, BAL
  - Biopsy
  - Therapeutic – removal of foreign body
- Diagnostic/therapeutic pleural tap
  - Microbiology M,C+S (including AAFBs)
  - Biochemistry – protein, glucose, LDH, pH, amylase
  - Cytology – malignant cells
  - Immunology – rheumatoid factor, ANA, complement
- CT-guided biopsy
- Pleural biopsy (mesothelioma)
- Kveim test (sarcoidosis)
- Fluoroscopy (diaphragmatic paralysis)
- EMG and nerve conduction studies – motor neurone disease, Guillain–Barré syndrome
- α_1-Antitrypsin levels
- Performance (exercise) testing, eg 6-minute walk test with oximetry

Swollen legs

➤ History of presenting complaint

Onset

When was the leg swelling first noticed?

Is it new or old?

Character

Has it affected one or both legs?

Where does the swelling extend to?

Is it at the bottom of your back and in your tummy?

Is there swelling of your arms too? (That is, is this generalised oedema?)

Associated symptoms

Is it painful? Is it pitting when you press it?

Is it hot or cold?

Has there been redness, exudates or skin changes? (Cellulitis)

Is there a history of knee arthritis or swelling behind the knee before onset? (Baker's cyst)

Are there any associated symptoms such as fever?

Precipitating factors

Has there been any injury to the leg/trauma/cellulitis?

Is there a history of an infected lesion, such as an ingrowing toenail/boil/ulcerating lesion?

Are there any symptoms suggestive of CCF? (Chest pain, breathlessness, syncope, palpitations (congenital heart disease, mitral valve disease), liver tenderness)

Are there any symptoms suggestive of renal disease? (Frothy urine?)

Are there any symptoms suggestive of liver disease? (Jaundice, bruising, pruritus)

Are there any symptoms of malabsorption? (Such as weight loss, steatorrhoea)

> ➤ *Risk factors for DVT*
>
> Prolonged immobility (surgery, plaster cast)
> Travel
> Previous DVT/PE
> Malignancy
> OCP

Is there any shortness of breath, chest pain, haemoptysis? (PE)

Are there any skin changes? (SLE, scleroderma cause pulmonary fibrosis → cor pulmonale)

Are there any abdominal masses or swellings? (Extrinsic venous compression) Are you currently pregnant?

Relieving factors

Does elevation of the legs help to reduce the swelling?

What do you think is wrong?

Ask about treatment already received? (Diuretics?)

➤ Past medical history

Is there any history of previous leg swelling?

Is there a past history of heart problems or valvular heart disease?

Have you had previous groin surgery? (Lymphoedema)

Have you had previous exposure to radiation/radiotherapy, or have you had a previous malignancy? (Lymphoedema)

Is there any history of previous DVTs, PEs or varicose vein operations?

Swollen legs

> Drug history

What medications do you take?

Do you take diuretics?

Have you started any new medications recently (eg amlodipine, nifedipine, fenfluramine, NSAIDs)?

Are you taking any anticoagulants for DVT prophylaxis?

Compliance, side-effect(s) of medication, OTC/herbal remedies, allergies. (What happens?)

> Social history

Do you use recreational drugs? (Nephrotic syndrome)

Have you been abroad? (Overseas travel history, tropical illnesses)

How do the symptoms interfere with your life? (Walking, working, sleeping)

Are you still able to put on shoes?

> Family history

Is there a family history of (lymph)oedema?

Is there a family history of DVTs/thrombophilia (eg PC/PS deficiency, factor V Leiden)?

Is there a family history of primary pulmonary hypertension?

> Differential diagnosis

Generalised disease

- **Right-sided heart failure**
- **Cor pulmonale**
- Hypoalbuminaemia
  - **Nephrotic syndrome**
  - **Liver failure**

- Malnutrition/malabsorption
- Protein-losing enteropathy
- Fluid overload (iatrogenic)
- Myxoedema

Localised disease

- Venous disease
  - **Deep venous thrombosis***
  - **Inferior vena cava (IVC) occlusion**
  - **External iliac vein compression by pelvic mass***
    - ➤ Tumours
    - ➤ Gravid uterus
  - **Venodilating drugs**
    - ➤ Calcium-channel antagonists (amlodipine, nifedipine, felodipine, verapamil, etc)
    - ➤ Vasodilators – minoxidil, diazoxide, hydralazine
    - ➤ Prostaglandin analogues (alprostadil)
    - ➤ NSAIDs (fluid retention)
- Lymphatic disease*
  - Primary lymphoedema (Milroy's syndrome)
  - Secondary (acquired) lymphoedema
    - ➤ Malignant infiltration
    - ➤ Post-inflammatory (fibrosis following cellulitis)
    - ➤ Post-irradiation fibrosis
    - ➤ Post-operative (radical surgery)
    - ➤ Filariasis infection
- Other important causes
  - **Compartment syndrome, trauma***
  - **Cellulitis***
  - **Ruptured Baker's cyst***
  - **Necrotising fasciitis***
  - Dependency
  - Disuse of limb (eg arthritis)*

* May cause *unilateral* swelling

> Investigations

Blood tests
- Haematology – FBC, clotting, D-dimers, ESR
  - Anaemia (anaemia of chronic disease)
  - Raised MCV (alcohol abuse)
  - Raised WCC (cellulitis)
  - Clotting (spontaneous haematomas)
  - D-dimers (DVT)
  - ESR (infection, inflammation)
- Biochemistry
  - U+Es (renal failure, hyponatraemia in CCF and cirrhosis)
  - Glucose (DM → cellulitis)
  - TFTs (myxoedema)
  - CRP (infection)
  - LFTs (liver failure)
  - Albumin (hypoalbuminaemia)

Microbiology
- Blood cultures (infection)
- Skin swab culture (cellulitis)

ECG
- Q waves (old MI)

Urinalysis
- Dipstick for protein, blood (renal failure)
- Glucose (DM → cellulitis)
- 24-hour urine collection for protein (nephrotic syndrome)

Radiology

- CXR
  - Cardiomegaly (CCF)
  - Pulmonary oedema (fluid overload)
- Limb X-ray
  - Fracture
  - Tumour
  - Gas (gas gangrene)
- Duplex Doppler USS (ileofemoral DVT, arteriovenous fistula)
- USS of swelling
  - Haematoma
  - Baker's cyst
  - Tumour
- Echocardiography
  - Valvular dysfunction
  - CCF

Further investigations

- USS or CT abdomen/pelvis
  - Pelvic mass causing extrinsic venous compression
  - IVC obstruction/compression
- Venography (DVT)
- Arteriography (arteriovenous fistula)
- Renal biopsy (nephritis)
- Bowel investigations (enteropathy)
- Lymphangiography (lymphoedema)
- Lymph node biopsy (infection, tumour)
- Thrombophilia screen (DVT)

Tinnitus

➤ History of presenting complaint

What is the problem exactly? Is it getting better/worse/staying the same over time?

SOCRATES

Site

If subjective, is it unilateral or bilateral? (former more likely to be associated with a serious disorder such as Ménière's disease, acoustic neuroma, cholesteatoma, vascular disease).

Onset

When do you hear the noise? In bed at night when it is most quiet?

Character

Is it a humming, buzzing, ringing, hissing, throbbing, roaring, whistling, beating, clicking, crackling, bubbling or musical noise? (NB voices need psychiatric referral)

Is it continuous or intermittent?

Is it pulsatile or non-pulsatile?

Is it subjective or objective? (Where is the noise coming from? Inside or outside your head?)

Can others hear what you are hearing at all? The latter is unusual but may indicate carotico-cavernous fistulae, glomus tumours, AVM, carotid stenosis, aneurysms, anaemia, a patent Eustachian tube or palatal myoclonus.

Associated symptoms

Do you have any vertigo or deafness? (Ménière's, acoustic neuroma, cholesteatoma, MS, basilar artery insufficiency/occlusion, brain stem tumours, syphilis)

Is there a sense of fullness of the ear? (Ménière's). Do you have earache, ear discharge, weakness of the face?

Precipitating factors

Do you normally suffer with ear wax? Is there any history of a FB being inserted into the ear?

Do you have any teeth, jaw or sinus problems?

Is there a history of trauma? (whiplash, concussion, trauma to the middle or inner ear?)

What is your occupation? Have you previously been exposed to loud noise either through work (road drillers, heavy artiliary), or outside work eg loud stereos, night clubs and hobbies (eg pigeon/clay shooting)?

Do you suffer from stress, fatigue?

Severity

What effect does it have on your life – work, sleep, mood, social activities, talking to people?

Are you able to concentrate on what you are doing?

Does it keep you awake at night or wake you up ever from your sleep?

Does it make you depressed? Has it ever been so bad that you've thought about taking your own life because of it?

What do you think is wrong?

Ask about treatment, if any, already received? eg Tinnitus maskers (white noise generators), betahistine, antidepressants. Have you tried a hearing aid?

Tinnitus

➤ Past medical history

Have you had previous head/whiplash injuries?

Have you had previous ear surgery, syringing, or middle ear infections?

Have you experienced any recent pressure changes? (deep sea/scuba diving, barotrauma, air flight)

Is there a history of HT, Paget's disease or renal failure?

Have you had previous consultations with audiologists and/or hearing therapists?

➤ Drug history

Do you take any medications?

Do you take any drugs that may precipitate tinnitus (aspirin overdose, loop diuretics, aminoglycosides such as gentamicin, tetracyclines, clindamycin, caffeine, TCAs, quinine)?

➤ Social history

Are there any current stressful life events (emotional, physical or behavioural) which may trigger tinnitus?

What is your occupation? (occupational exposures – loud noise), exercise capacity, lifestyle limitations due to disease.

Psychosocial history – Isolation, divorce, bereavement, redundancy.

Have you taken time off work? How much?

How do the symptoms interfere with your life (walking, working, sleeping)?

What is extent of your disability?

➤ Family history

Is there a FHx of otosclerosis?

➤ Differential diagnosis

Local

- **Ear wax**
- **Presbyacusis**
- **Ménière's disease**
- **Noise-induced deafness**
- Otitis media
- Otosclerosis
- Aneurysms/AVMs and fistulae
- Bruits
- **Tumours**
  - **Acoustic neuroma**
  - **Glomus jugulare tumour**
  - **Chemodectoma**
  - **Nasopharyngeal carcinoma**
- Trauma (head injury)
  - Basal skull fracture
- Impacted wisdom teeth
- Temporomandibular joint dysfunction
- Palatal myoclonus

General

- Fever of any cause
- Cardiovascular
  - Hypertension
  - CCF
  - Atherosclerosis
- Renal failure (hypertension)
- Haematological
  - Anaemia
  - Raised viscosity
- Neurological
  - MS
  - Neuropathy
- Paget's disease

- **Drugs**
  - **Aspirin**
  - **Quinine**
  - **Beta-blockers**
  - **Ototoxic drugs**
    - ➤ **Aminoglycosides**
    - ➤ **Loop diuretics**
  - **Alcohol abuse**

➤ Investigations

Blood tests
- Haematology: FBC
  - anaemia
  - MCV (alcohol)
- Biochemistry:
  - U+Es (renal failure)
  - LFTs (alcohol abuse)
  - Salicylate levels

Age appropriate hearing test/audiometry (to assess hearing loss objectively)

Impedance tympanometry

Radiology
- MRI:
  - Acoustic neuroma
  - AVMs

Further investigations
- **Skull X-ray** (Paget's disease, head injury)
- **Alkaline phosphatase** (Paget's disease)
- **Cerebral angiography** (aneurysms, AVMs, fistulae)
- **Carotid Dopplers** (carotid stenosis, chemodectoma)

Tremor and movement disorders

➤ History of presenting complaint

Site

Is it unilateral or bilateral?

What is the exact problem?

Where is the movement/tremor most of a problem? (hands, feet, head, jaw, voice, tongue etc)

Has anyone else noticed it apart from yourself?

Onset

Was onset gradual or sudden?

Over what time period (hours, days, weeks, years)?

Does it seem to be getting worse, better or staying the same?

How often does it occur?

Is it all the time, or does it occur intermittently? If the latter, what precipitates it?

Character

What is the movement like? (tremor, jerks etc), slow vs fast?

Do you have any control over it? (involuntary vs voluntary)

Do you have difficulty in starting/initiating movement from rest or stopping?

Do you have difficulty rising from a chair?

What are you like once you get going?

Have your movements slowed down? (bradykinesia)

Do you ever find yourself being stuck to the floor?

Do you have difficulty getting into and out of the bath?

How long does this take you?

Associated symptoms

What have others close to you noticed about you recently?

Do your movements feel stiff (rigidity)? Do you suffer from muscle fatigue? Have you noticed any changes in your walking, gait or posture?

What about your voice – has anyone close to you noticed a change in volume (quieter?) or character (monotonous?) (PD, cerebellar)?

Has your handwriting changed character in any way? Is it becoming more difficult to read?

Are you still able to smile and make appropriate facial expressions? Is this is because you are depressed or unable to make appropriate facial expressions?

Do you have difficulty swallowing, or have you found drooling from the mouth to be a problem?

Is your blinking affected?

Do you suffer from urinary/faecal incontinence?

Is rolling over in bed difficult? Do you and your wife/ husband sometimes find yourselves fighting over the bed covers at night?

Do you ever have to wake up your partner, or does your partner ever wake up at night, to assist you in turning over in bed?

Do you snore at all at night? (respiratory stridor is characteristic of multiple system atrophy)

Do you get dizzy when you stand up? (autonomic-neuropathy – Shy–Drager syndrome)

Have you noticed problems looking up or down? (progressive supranuclear palsy)

Have you become more forgetful? (Lewy body dementia)

Do you have any skin changes (seborrhoea – PD)

Is depression a problem or do you feel low at times?

Do you suffer from vertigo, balance problems, or problems with coordination? (cerebellar pathology)

Are there any features of hyperthyroidism – diarrhoea, increased appetite, weight loss, palpitations, eye changes, heat intolerance, neck lumps?

Are you generally an anxious person?

Precipitating factors

When does it occur and when is it worst? (at rest when relaxed, when reaching out to fetch something (ie during movement), when your hands are held outstretched in front of you (ie in a sustained position or against gravity as when engaging in activities)

Does the tremor affect your arms, hands, (which side is worse? Are you left or right handed?), jaw, head (titubation-seen in BET), feet, eyelids (blepharospasm), tongue (BET) or voice (what happens to your voice when you speak in front of a large audience? If voice is primarily affected, anxiety or BET is more likely).

If you are anxious, emotionally stressed or fatigued what effect does this have on the tremor?

What happens to the movement when you close your eyes?

Does gripping an object (eg when holding a glass) have any effect on the tremor? Give examples of difficulty such as holding drinks, bringing a glass of fluid to their mouth, passing a teacup and saucer to someone, during writing etc.

Does the cold affect it (shivering?)

Relieving factors

What effect does alcohol have on the movement? What about beta-blockers? Does it respond to L-DOPA?

Does relaxation have any effect on the tremor?

What helps you to get going (any sensory cues)? What happens when you walk through doorways?

Do you find you walk better on flat or uneven ground?

What effect does concentrating on the movement have?

What happens at night when you are asleep? Do the movements persist during sleep (myoclonus) or do they disappear (tremors, chorea)? (dystonias may or may not persist during sleep)

Severity

What effect does it have on your quality of life?

What bothers you most about the tremor? What are your main concerns? The fact that there may be a serious underlying illness (such as Parkinson's disease), or the fact that others notice it?

What do you think is wrong?

Ask about treatment, if any, already received?

➤ Past medical history

Are there any previous psychiatric or neurological problems?

Is there a history of epilepsy or jaundice (Wilson's disease → metabolic flap)

Have you had rheumatic fever? (Sydenham's chorea)

Have you ever had a stroke? (hemiballismus)

Is there a history of respiratory/renal/liver disease? (metabolic flap)

Do you suffer from asthma? (salbutamol can cause a tremor, also in asthma beta-blockers, as a treatment option for tremor, are contraindicated as they may worsen bronchospasm)

➤ Drug history

Do you take any medications that may cause movement disorders such as: caffeine, antipsychotics, metoclopramide, prochlorperazine, haloperidol, lithium, phenytoin, valproate, ciclosporin, salbutamol, levodopa?

➤ Social history

Do you smoke? How much and for how long? (nicotine withdrawal)

Do you drink alcohol? (BET, cerebellar problems, alcohol withdrawal)

Do you use recreational drugs? (drug withdrawal, MPTP)

Functional status – what does it stop you doing? Does it stop you performing skilled movements? Are you able to complete/manage

Tremor and movement disorders

everyday tasks because of it? For example, are you able to dress yourself? Undo buttons? Open jars? Tie your shoes? Clean your teeth? Bathe/shower yourself? Cook yourself? Are you able to feed yourself? Do you ever spill food or drink over yourself? Does it affect your ability to drive? Can you still write legibly?

How are you on your feet?

How do you get around (unaided or with the use of a walking aid such as a stick or zimmer frame?)

Do you suffer from episodes of frequent falling? (PD, progressive supranuclear palsy)?

What help do you have at home?

What sort of place do you live in?

Can you continue to roll pastry, beat eggs, do the ironing, peel potatoes, wring out washing, use a screwdriver, saw or hammer effectively?

What impact does the disease have on your family?

What is your occupation? (have you been exposed to mercury?), lifestyle limitations due to disease (eg not being able to paint or write any more)

Have you taken time off work? How much?

How far can you usually walk, what stops you?

How do the symptoms interfere with your life (walking, working, sleeping)?

> # Family history

Is there a FHx of tremor or movement disorders? (NB: One third of patients with BET have a positive FHx).

Is there a FHx of Huntington's, Wilson's, Parkinson's diseases, myoclonus/Creutzfeldt–Jakob disease?

Is there any consanguinity? Draw a family tree.

Differentiating a benign essential tremor from a parkinsonian tremor on the basis of the history

Benign essential tremor (BET)	Parkinsonian tremor
Familial (autosomal dominant inheritance) Primarily postural tremor Higher frequency tremor (10 Hz) Relieved by beta-blockers Relieved by alcohol Tends to spare lower limbs Head often involved (titubation) Voice often involved	Primarily resting tremor Lower frequency tremor (4–6 Hz) Involves lower limbs and jaw more often than BET L-DOPA responsive (idiopathic Parkinson's disease) Other features of parkinsonism usually present (cogwheeling, leadpipe rigidity, bradykinesia, postural instability)

Teasing apart the three main types of tremor

	Benign essential (action/postural) (~10 Hz)	Parkinsonian (~5 Hz)	Intention (cerebellar) (~5 Hz)
Rest	–	+ +	–
Posture	+ +	+	+
Movement	+	–	+ +

➤ Differential diagnosis

Tremor

Postural tremor

- Benign essential tremor (~ 10 Hz)

Action tremor

- Cerebellar intention tremor (3–5 Hz)

Resting tremor

- **Parkinsonism** (4–6 Hz):
  - Neurodegeneration
    - ➤ Parkinson's disease
    - ➤ Multiple system atrophy
    - ➤ Supranuclear palsy
  - Neuroleptics
    - ➤ Metoclopramide
    - ➤ Prochlorperazine
    - ➤ Haloperidol
  - Post-encephalitis
  - Lewy body dementia
- Exaggerated physiological tremor (6–12 Hz):
  - Thyrotoxicosis
  - Phaeochromocytoma
  - Drug-induced: salbutamol, caffeine, alcohol, lithium, phenytoin, ciclosporin
  - Drug withdrawal: opiates, benzodiazepines, alcohol
  - Metabolic flap: hepatic/uraemic encephalopathy, CO_2 retention
  - Hypoglycaemia
  - Anxiety
  - Exercise
- Wilson's disease
- Tertiary syphilis
- Hysteria

Other involuntary movements

Chorea

- **Huntington's disease**
- Sydenham's chorea
- Wilson's disease
- Drugs:
  - Oral contraception
  - L-dopa
  - Antipsychotics

- Pregnancy (chorea gravidarum)
- Thyrotoxicosis
- SLE
- Hyperviscosity

Dystonia

- Idiopathic
  - Writer's cramp
  - Spasmodic torticollis
- Drugs: antipsychotics, antiemetics, anticonvulsants
- Wilson's disease

Myoclonus

- Congenital
- Physiological: myoclonic jerks in sleep
- Acute metabolic encephalopathy
- Myoclonic epilepsy
- Creutzfeldt–Jakob disease
- Alzheimer's disease
- Lysosomal storage diseases, eg Gaucher's, Tay–Sachs disease

➤ Investigations

Blood tests

- Haematology – FBC
  - Macrocytosis (alcohol)
- Biochemistry
  - U+Es (uraemic flap)
  - TFTs (hyperthyroid tremor, hypothyroidism → cerebellar dysfunction)
  - Glucose (hypoglycaemia)
  - Serum caeruloplasmin/copper (Wilson's disease)
  - CRP (infection)
  - LFTs (alcohol abuse, liver failure, Wilson's disease)
- Arterial blood gas (carbon dioxide retention)

Radiology

- CT/MRI head:
  - Cerebellar space-occupying lesion
  - Demyelination
  - Other areas of neurodegeneration

Further investigations

- Lumbar puncture (MS, meningoencephalitis)
- Visually evoked potentials (MS)
- Syphilis serology
- Genetic (trinucleotide repeat) studies (Huntington's disease)
- PET scan (uptake abnormalities in basal ganglia in Parkinson's)

Tremor and movement disorders

Upper gastrointestinal bleeding

➤ History of presenting complaint

First confirm that it is *true* haematemesis, rather than coughed-up blood (haemoptysis), or blood from the upper respiratory passages which the patient has swallowed and subsequently vomited, so-called 'pseudohaematemesis'. (Ask about previous nosebleeds and coughing up of any blood.)

SOCRATES

Onset

When did it start? Is this the first time?

Character

Has the patient been vomiting fresh blood or coffee-grounds? Are there any clots?

How much, how many times, and how long does it last for? How much blood have you vomited? (In cupfuls)

Does the first vomit contain blood or only subsequent ones? (Mallory–Weiss tear)

Was the episode preceded by intense retching?

Is the bleed effortless? (Varices)

Associated symptoms

Has there been any indigestion, heartburn, acid reflux, dysphagia or abdominal pain? (Latter – PUD)

Is there any odynophagia? (Oesophagitis)

Do you think you have jaundice? (Chronic liver disease)

Is there any blood loss from the back passage or melaena? Is blood mixed in with the stool or separate from it? Is blood present on the toilet paper?

Is there any change in bowel habit? Is there any pain on defecation? Is there any mucus? Is there any diarrhoea?

Do you feel faint or dizzy, especially with sitting/standing upright? Is there any sweating, palpitations, weakness, pallor, breathlessness? (Features of shock)

Are there any features of malignancy – weight loss, dysphagia, anorexia, malaise, lethargy?

Are there any symptoms suggestive of chronic anaemia – reduced exercise tolerance, fatigue, angina/chest pain, breathlessness, etc?

Precipitating factors

> ➤ *PUD risk factors*

NSAIDs
Smoking
Corticosteroids
Stress
Alcohol
Biliary reflux

Relieving factors

Do you get relief from antacids?

What do you think is wrong?

Ask about treatment already received.

> Past medical history

Is there a history of GI blood loss and its causes, ulcers, anaemia, bleeding tendency, liver disease?

Is there a history of bowel surgery (eg leading to biliary reflux, which is a risk factor for PUD), AAA repairs, or bleeding disorders?

Is there a past history of heart, lung, liver or renal disease, or malignancy? (Rockall scoring)

> Drug history

What medications do you take?

- NSAIDs
- Warfarin
- Steroids
- Iron tablets (produces black stools)

Alcohol

PPIs

Compliance, side-effect(s) of medication, OTC/herbal remedies, allergies. (What happens?)

> Social history

Do you smoke? How much and for how long?

How much alcohol do you drink? (Gastritis, PUD, varices)

Do you use recreational drugs?

Have you been abroad? (Overseas travel history, tropical illnesses)

Vaccinations? (Such as typhoid, hepatitis)

> Family history

Is there a family history of colitis, bowel malignancy, or rare hereditary bleeding conditions such as Osler–Weber–Rendu syndrome?

Is there any consanguinity? *Draw a family tree.*

➤ Differential diagnosis

General

- Bleeding diatheses
  - Anticoagulation therapy
  - Haemophilia
  - Hereditary haemorrhagic telangiectasia (Osler–Weber–Rendu disease)
- Exclude **pseudohaematemesis** (vomiting of swallowed blood from a nasal/pharyngeal haemorrhage)

Local

Common

- **Bleeding duodenal/gastric (peptic) ulcer**
- **Gastro-oesophageal varices**
- **Erosive oesophagogastritis**
- **Mallory–Weiss tear**
- **Drug-related**
  - NSAIDs
  - Anticoagulants
  - Steroids
  - Thrombolytics
  - Alcohol
- Oesophageal/gastric tumours (benign/malignant)

Rare

- Aorto-duodenal fistula
  - Haemobilia
  - Angiodysplasia
  - Dieulafoy's lesion (gastric vascular malformation)

➤ Investigations

Blood tests

- Haematology – FBC, clotting, ESR, cross-match/G+S
  - Anaemia (severe bleed, carcinoma, blood dyscrasias)
  - MCV (alcohol)
  - Clotting (liver disease, bleeding diatheses)
  - ESR (connective tissue disease, vasculitides, eg PAN)
  - Cross-match, G+S (severe bleed)
- Biochemistry
  - U+Es (urea disproportionately raised compared with creatinine, indicating a protein load of fresh blood within the gut as well as pre-renal failure, hyperkalaemia from absorbed blood, Rockall scoring)
  - LFTs (liver disease, varices, haemobilia, Rockall scoring)
  - Glucose (liver disease)
  - Amylase

ECG

- Cardiac ischaemia if massive blood loss
- Co-morbid cardiac disease (Rockall scoring)

Faecal occult blood three times

OGD ± biopsies and *Helicobacter pylori* testing

- Diagnostic – varices, bleeding PUD, erosive oesophagogastritis, Mallory–Weiss tear, carcinoma
- Therapeutic – variceal banding/sclerotherapy, injection with adrenaline/cautery of actively bleeding peptic ulcer
- Surveillance – variceal size, whether healing of gastric ulcer has taken place (ie exclude gastric malignancy)
- Prognostic (Rockall scoring) – stigmata of recent haemorrhage

Radiology

- (Erect) CXR
  - Aspiration of vomitus
  - Perforation of viscus (eg ruptured oesophagus)
  - Co-morbidities (Rockall scoring)
- USS abdomen
  - Liver cirrhosis
  - Portal hypertension
  - AAA
- Barium swallow
  - Malignancy
- CT thorax, abdomen, pelvis
  - Staging of carcinoma
  - Aortic graft infection

Further investigations

- Angiography (vascular malformations)

Vaginal bleeding

➤ History of presenting complaint

Site

Confirm it is vaginal rather than urethral or rectal bleeding.

Onset

Was it expected? (Menses)

When did it start and was the onset sudden or gradual? What has the duration been?

When was the first day of your last menstrual period? Was it on time?

When was your last withdrawal bleed? (OCP) Is there any chance that you could be pregnant? Are you pre- or post-menopausal?

Character

What is the timing and relationship to the menstrual cycle?

What is the frequency?

What is the colour?

What is the odour?

What is the consistency?

What is the volume?

Does it feel like a period to you, with the usual period-type symptoms?

Is the bleeding regular/cyclical/catamenial or irregular? (Regular = menses, ovulatory bleeding, endometriosis) Is the bleeding continuous or intermittent? Do you keep a menstrual diary?

What is the volume of blood loss? (Spotting, flooding)

What is the colour of blood loss? (Fresh red vs prune juice)

Character of menses:

- Was the last period normal in volume and duration?
- Are your cycles normally regular or irregular?

- What is your normal duration from one period to the next?
- What is your normal duration of bleeding?
- Do you normally suffer from heavy (menorrhagia) or painful periods (dysmenorrhoea)?
- Has the bleeding ± pain been worse than a normal period?

Is the bleeding IMB/PCB/PMB?

Does the bleeding occur mid-cycle?

Have products of conception been seen? (Clots may be mistaken for products)

Do you pass clots? How big are they? Do you have to wear pads/ sanitary wear? How many times do you have to change the pads/ tampons daily? Is there a need for double protection? What effect does it have on the quality of your life?

Associated symptoms

Is there any pain? What came first, the bleeding or the pain? (If pain is first, ectopic is more likely; if bleeding is first, miscarriage is more likely)

Is there any associated dyspareunia? (Superficial or deep) Is there any itching of the vulva? (Pruritus vulvae)

Is there any acne or hirsutism? (PCOS)

Is there any other vaginal discharge? What is the timing and relationship to the menstrual cycle? What is the frequency? What is the colour? What is the odour? What is the consistency? Is there any blood mixed in with the discharge? What is the volume? Does your partner have discharge as well?

Is there any abdominal/period/shoulder-tip pain?

Where exactly is the pain?

What was the onset like? (Sudden vs gradual)

Is it constant?

Are there any contractions or is it colicky?

Is it cyclical? Is there any associated fever? (PID)

Do you suffer from abdominal swelling or bloating? (Blood!, ovarian carcinoma, fibroids, ascites)

Are there any urinary symptoms? (Frequency, urgency, urge incontinence, dysuria, retention, haematuria) *Or rectal symptoms?* (Change in bowel habit, diarrhoea, painful defecation, rectal bleeding as a result of pelvic masses causing extrinsic compression, pelvic blood, PID, endometriomas)

Are there any features of thyroid dysfunction, especially hypothyroidism? (Weight gain, cold intolerance, constipation, hirsutism)

Precipitating factors

Is there a history of foreign body insertion?

Severity

Are there any features of shock (concealed haemorrhage) – Do you feel dizzy when you stand up? Are you thirsty? Is there flooding? (For example, in the bed)

Are there any features of anaemia from the bleeding, such as chest pain, palpitations, fatigue, pallor?

Pregnancy

Are you pregnant?

How many weeks into pregnancy are you?

> ➤ *Risk factors for ectopic pregnancy*

Prior PID

Previous IUCD use

Previous infertility

Assisted fertilisation (IVF/GIFT treatment)

Progesterone-only pill

Endometriosis

Prior ectopic pregnancy

Smoking

Previous abdominal/pelvic surgery (adhesions)

Congenital malformations

Have you encountered any problems so far? (For example on USS)

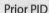

What do you think is wrong?

Ask about treatment, if any, already received.

➤ Past medical history

Review of gynaecological history

Have you had previous bleeding and pain?

When did your periods start? (Age of menarche)

When did your periods stop? (Age of menopause)

When was your last Pap smear? Was it normal?

Have you ever suffered from pelvic inflammatory disease?

Is there a history of hypertension/DM? (Risk factors for endometrial carcinoma)

Is there a history of breast carcinoma? (*BRCA* gene is associated with ovarian carcinoma; tamoxifen increases risk of endometrial carcinoma)

Is there a history of infertility?

Have you had any previous operations?

Review of obstetric history

How many children have you had? (Parity) When did you have them?

Did you have any antenatal problems?

What was the mode of delivery each time and were there any associated complications?

Did you reach full term?

Were there any premature deliveries?

What was the gestation outcome? (And weights of the babies)

Were any problems encountered in the puerperium?

Have you had any terminations and/or miscarriages – at what stage, why and how?

Have you had difficulty conceiving?

➤ Drug history

Do you take any medications?

What contraception are you using? (OCP, IUCD) Are you happy with it? What have you tried previously?

Are you on the pill – which type? Do you take injections? (Depo-Provera®)

Are you on HRT? If so, which type? (Unopposed oestrogen or combined oestrogen and progesterone?)

Do you take or have you ever taken tamoxifen? (Increases risk of endometrial carcinoma)

Have you missed doses of your pill? Have you had recent D+V? Have you been on recent antibiotic therapy?

Are you currently in the first few months of treatment with the pill? (Breakthrough bleeding with OCPs)

Do you take anticoagulants?

Compliance, side-effect(s) of medication, OTC/herbal remedies, allergies. (What happens?)

➤ Social history

Do you smoke? (Risk factor for ectopic) How much and for how long?

Have you taken time off work? How much?

Sexual history – are you sexually active? (PID, STIs, including HPV-related cervical carcinoma) Is your partner healthy?

How do the symptoms interfere with your life? (Walking, sleeping)

➤ Family history

Is there a family history of miscarriages, gynaecological carcinoma or ectopic pregnancies?

Is there a FHx of breast carcinoma? (*BRCA* gene and ovarian carcinoma)

Is there a family history of vWD?

➤ Differential diagnosis

General causes

- Bleeding diatheses – coagulopathies, thrombocytopenia, leukaemias, vWD, anticoagulation therapy
- Thyroid dysfunction (especially hypothyroidism)

Gynaecological causes

- Physiological – normal menses
- **Pregnancy-related** (early pregnancy)
- Ovulatory bleed (associated with mittelschmerz)
- Anovulation – perimenopause/perimenarche/PCOS
- Dysfunctional uterine bleeding
- **Drug-related breakthrough bleeding** – OCP, Depo-Provera®, HRT
- Trauma – IUCD, foreign bodies (eg pessaries)
- **Ectopic pregnancy**
- Ovarian cyst accident (rupture, haemorrhage, torsion)
- Inflammation – cervicitis, vaginitis (post-menopausal atrophic), endometritis
- **PID**
- Cystic glandular hyperplasia (metropathia haemorrhagica)
- Neoplasia
  - Benign
    - ➤ **Submucosal/polypoid uterine fibroids**
    - ➤ **Cervical/endometrial polyps**
    - ➤ **Cervical ectropion/erosion**
    - ➤ **Endometriosis**
    - ➤ **Hydatidiform mole** (partial/complete)
  - Malignant
    - ➤ **Endometrial**
    - ➤ **Cervix**
    - ➤ **Vulva**
    - ➤ **Ovarian**
    - ➤ **Fallopian tube**
    - ➤ **Choriocarcinoma**

Consider these additional causes during pregnancy:

- **Miscarriage**
- **Placental abruption**
- **Placenta praevia**

➤ Investigations

Blood tests

- Haematology – FBC, clotting, ESR, cross-match/G+S
  - Anaemia (blood loss)
  - Raised WCC (PID)
  - Thrombocytopenia (bleeding diatheses)
  - Clotting (bleeding diatheses, eg vWD)
  - ESR (malignancy, infection, inflammation)
  - Cross-match/G+S (severe bleed)
- Biochemistry
  - U+Es (renal function)
  - TFTs (thyroid dysfunction)
  - CRP (infection)
  - FSH/LH (premature menopause)
  - Tumour markers
  - β-hCG (ectopic, trophoblastic disease)
  - CA 125 (ovarian carcinoma)

Microbiology

- High vaginal swab/endocervical swab (PID, cervicitis)

Urinalysis

- Pus cells, nitrites, protein, M,C+S (UTI)
- β-hCG (ectopic, trophoblastic disease)

Speculum examination ± cervical smear

Vaginal bleeding

Radiology

- Pelvic (transvaginal) USS (uterine/ovarian pathology)
  - Anembryonic uterus, fluid in the cul-de-sac, adnexal mass (ectopic)
  - Foreign body
  - Ovarian cysts/mass
  - Uterine fibroids
  - Endometrial thickening
  - Tubo-ovarian abscess (PID)
  - Hydatidiform mole
  - Establish nature of problem in pregnancy
- CT/MRI thorax, abdomen, pelvis (metastases and staging)

Further investigations

- Colposcopy ± biopsy (cervical carcinoma and other cervical pathology)
  - Punch biopsy
  - Cone biopsy
  - Large loop excision of transformation zone
- Endometrial sampling (endometrial carcinoma) by:
  - Pipelle biopsy
  - Hysteroscopy
  - Dilatation and curettage (D+C)
- Hysteroscopy (endometrial pathology)
- Examination under anaesthetic (EUA)
- Diagnostic laparoscopy ± biopsy (pelvic visualisation in pelvic disease, PID, endometriosis, ectopic pregnancy and masses)

Visual loss (acute and chronic)

➤ History of presenting complaint

Is the visual loss unilateral/monocular or bilateral/binocular?

Is it complete or incomplete?

SOCRATES

Onset

Was it sudden or gradual?

Character

Is the problem primarily a loss of part/whole of the visual field, loss of visual acuity, blurring of vision, double vision, loss of colour vision, or positive phenomena?

Which particular area of the visual field is affected?

Period over which it lasted? Is it fleeting? (Emboli, migraine, raised ICP) Or prolonged? (Anterior ischaemic optic neuropathy, optic neuritis, retinal artery occlusion, retinal vein occlusion, vitreous haemorrhage, retinal detachment)

Is it painful? Is it worse with eye movement? Is there a headache with it?

Do you wear glasses/contact lenses? When? Are you short-sighted or long-sighted? Do you need to wear reading glasses? When were your eyes last tested?

When is it worst? (At night = retinitis pigmentosa, cataracts)

Associated symptoms

Are there any other associated symptoms? (Flashing lights and shapes/ scintillations/zigzag lines, floaters, coloured haloes, aura of migraine, tunnel vision, loss of colour vision, double vision?)

Is the eye red?

Is there any exudate? (Presence, amount, colour)

Is the eye watering? (Cluster headaches, iritis, keratitis)

Is there any headache or facial pain – is this unilateral or bilateral?

Is there any pain on eating (jaw claudication), proximal muscle weakness, facial pain, or tenderness over the superficial temporal artery?

Are there any associated neurological symptoms, such as unilateral weakness, clumsiness, numbness or paraesthesia?

Are there any systemic symptoms, such as fever, malaise, vomiting, arthralgia, rashes or headache?

Is there any photophobia?

Are there any symptoms of raised ICP – Are the headaches worse with straining, sneezing or coughing? When are they worst? (In the morning?) Is there associated nausea, vomiting or drowsiness?

Do you have difficulty driving at night? Why? Do car headlights bother you at all? Do you suffer from glare? Has your glasses prescription changed recently? Do you no longer require glasses for reading? (Cataracts)

Do you have difficulty reading, eating, watching TV? Can you see the whole of people's faces or are there holes/bits missing? When you read, are the words on the page distorted in any way? How? (Macular degeneration)

Can you see where you are going? Do you ever bump into things? Can you see to go up/down stairs? (Visual field defects)

Is there a history of foreign body insertion or trauma to the head or eye?

Cardiovascular risk factors (amaurosis fugax, central retinal artery/vein occlusion) – see Chest pain.

What do you think is wrong?

Ask about treatment, if any, already received.

➤ Past medical history

Is there a history of eye problems?

Have you had herpes infection previously on your face? (Especially in the distribution of the ophthalmic division of the trigeminal nerve (Va), such as vesicles on the tip of the nose – Hutchinson's sign – this may subsequently involve the eye)

Is there a history of retinal detachment?

Do you wear contact lenses? Do these cause you any problems?

Is there a history of thyroid eye disease?

Have you had recent cataract surgery?

Have you had laser surgery on your eyes?

Is there any significant past medical history, such as hypertension, IHD, DM (insulin- or non-insulin-dependent?), glaucoma, MS, other risk factors for strokes/TIAs, migraine, or connective tissue disorders?

➤ Drug history

Do you take any medications, such as eye drops for glaucoma?

Are you taking steroids? (Cataracts)

Compliance, side-effect(s) of medication, OTC/herbal remedies, allergies. (What happens?)

➤ Social history

Do you smoke?

Do you consume much alcohol?

Have you been exposed to radiation? (Cataracts)

Have you been abroad? (Overseas travel history, tropical illnesses)

Have you taken time off work? How much?

How do the symptoms interfere with your life? (Walking, working, sleeping)

What is the extent of your visual disability?

Are you registered blind now?

Do you have adaptations at home to help with your visual disability?

Do you have a guide dog? Have you thought about getting one?

➤ Family history

Is there a family history of glaucoma or retinitis pigmentosa?

Is there any consanguinity? *Draw a family tree.*

➤ Differential diagnosis

Sudden loss of vision

Painful and prolonged

- **Acute angle-closure glaucoma**
- **Optic neuritis**
- **Giant cell arteritis**
- **Anterior uveitis (iritis)**
- **Orbital cellulitis**
- **Endophthalmitis**

Painless and fleeting

- **Amaurosis fugax**
- Migraine*
- **Raised ICP** (papilloedema)*

Painless and prolonged

- **Retinal detachment**
- **Vitreous haemorrhage** (especially DM)
- **Retinal artery occlusion**
- **Retinal vein occlusion**
- **Anterior ischaemic optic neuropathy**
- Occipital lobe infarct*

* Tend to be bilateral (unless *retinal* migraine)

Gradual loss of vision

Congenital

- **Retinitis pigmentosa**

Acquired

- **Refractive errors**
- **Cataracts**
- **Age-related macular degeneration**
- **Diabetic retinopathy/maculopathy**
- **Chronic glaucoma**
- Hypertensive retinopathy
- Optic nerve compression
- Intraorbital/intracranial space-occupying lesion

➤ Investigations

Blood tests

- Haematology – FBC, ESR
  - Raised Hb (polycythaemia rubra vera → hyperviscosity syndrome → retinal vein occlusion)
  - Raised WCC (infection)
  - ESR (giant cell arteritis)
- Biochemistry
  - U+Es (diabetic nephropathy – associated with retinopathy)
  - Glucose (diabetes mellitus)
  - HbA_{1c} (glycaemic control)
  - CRP (infection, giant cell arteritis)

Urine dipstick

- Glucose (diabetes mellitus)

Direct/indirect fundoscopy

Slit lamp examination

Tonometry (glaucoma)

Perimetry (visual field analysis)

Further investigations

- Temporal artery biopsy (giant cell arteritis)
- Fluorescein angiography (diabetic retinopathy, retinal artery/vein occlusion)
- Skull X-ray (Paget's disease)
- CT head (ischaemia, space-occupying lesion)
- MRI head (demyelination)
- Retinal/posterior-pole USS (useful in presence of cataract or vitreous haemorrhage to identify treatable retinal causes of visual loss)
- Visually evoked potentials (MS)
- Lumbar puncture (MS)
- Lipids (modifiable risk factor for retinal artery/vein occlusion)
- Carotid Doppler (carotid stenosis)
- ECG and echocardiogram (as source of embolus for retinal artery occlusion)

Visual loss (acute and chronic)

Vomiting

➤ History of presenting complaint

First try to establish what the patient actually means by vomiting – retching, nausea, actual vomitus?

When did the vomiting start?

What were you doing when the vomiting started?

Were you well before the vomiting started?

SOCRATES

Onset

How quickly did it come on? (Instantaneous, seconds, over minutes, hours)

Duration?

Have you ever had it before?

Character

What did you vomit? (Altered food, blood (bright-red or altered), coffee grounds?

Is it extremely watery?

Is there undigested/recently-eaten, recognisable food in it? (Fresh or old food)

Is it bile-stained? Faeculent?

How much did you vomit? (In cupfuls) Is it projectile in nature? (Gastric outflow obstruction, rasied ICP, acute pancreatitis, severe GORD)

What about the taste and smell of the vomitus?

Associated symptoms

Are you managing to drink and keep any fluids down?

What else did you notice? (Any associated abdominal pain, headache, drowsiness, fits (ICP), other pains, chest pain (could be MI or Boerhaave's), testicular pain (torsion), iritis (Crohn's disease), diarrhoea, abdominal distension, constipation, sweating/fever, jaundice, reduced appetite/weight loss, rash, arthralgia or symptoms of anaemia (fatigue, malaise, breathlessness, chest pain)?)

Are there any symptoms of fluid depletion – faintness, dizziness on standing up?

Do you have vertigo, hearing loss or tinnitus? *Are there any symptoms of neurological disease*, such as aura or headaches? (Migraine, ICP)

Timing

When does the vomiting occur and how frequently? Do you get it at night?

How long does it occur for? At what time of day does it occur? Is it related to meal times? Does it occur in the early morning? (Pregnancy, ICP, alcoholism) Or in the late evening? Is it straight after eating, or an hour or more after eating? (Former suggests PUD, gastric carcinoma; latter is characteristic of gastric outflow obstruction)

Is it associated with bouts of coughing?

How quickly did it come on? Is it heralded by nausea, or does it occur without warning? (Latter indicates ICP or gastric outflow obstruction)

When you are not vomiting, does the nausea persist?

Precipitating factors

What precipitated it? Is it related to food or medications? (Movement, eating, hospital food)

Have you eaten any unusual foods or been abroad recently?

Have you eaten in a restaurant recently? (If yes, where and the timing and details of the type of food that was eaten are important for the diagnosis)

Has there been any contact with others with diarrhoea and vomiting?

Relieving factors

Do you have dyspepsia or abdominal pain? (Heartburn) Does vomiting relieve the symptoms? (Indicates PUD)

Severity

Severity of episodes and how life has been affected.

Is there any possibility of pregnancy, or overdose/intoxication of drugs/alcohol?

Are there any features of bowel obstruction – abdominal distension, failure to pass faeces and, more importantly, failure to pass flatus (absolute constipation), colicky abdominal pain? Do you have any hernias?

What do you think is wrong?

Ask about treatment already received? (Such as loperamide)

➤ Past medical history

MITJTHREADS

Are you diabetic?

Is there a history of previous vomiting?

Is there a history of known GI disease, eg IBD, pancreatitis, bowel malignancy?

Has there been previous abdominal and bowel surgery?

Is there a history of previous episodes of bowel obstruction due to, for example, adhesions?

Is there a history of ingestion of emetic medications? (Especially chemotherapy, opiates and radiotherapy)

Is there a history of bulimia/anorexia, with abuse of emetics?

Is there a history of migraines or motion sickness?

Is there a history of renal failure or alcohol misuse?

Have you had any recent chest infections? (Aspiration)

➤ Drug history

Are you taking any drugs which may have precipitated the vomiting? (Chemotherapy, opiates, NSAIDs, aspirin)

➤ Social history

Do you smoke? How much?

Do you drink much alcohol? How much?

Do you use recreational drugs?

Have you been abroad? (Overseas travel history, tropical illnesses)

Vaccinations? (Such as typhoid, hepatitis)

➤ Family history

Is there a family history of IBD or gut malignancy?

➤ Differential diagnosis

GI pathology

- Obstruction
  - **Small/large bowel obstruction**
  - **Pyloric stenosis**
- Inflammation
  - **Appendicitis**
  - **Biliary colic, cholecystitis**
  - **Peptic ulcer disease**
  - **Pancreatitis**
  - **Peritonitis**
- Infective – **gastroenteritis**, eg
  - *Salmonella*
  - *Campylobacter*

Metabolic

- **Pregnancy**
- Uraemia
- **Diabetic ketoacidosis**
- **Hypercalcaemia**
- Addison's

Vomiting

Drugs

- **Alcohol**
- **Opioids**
- Antibiotics
- NSAIDs
- Poisons – arsenic, iron
- Digoxin
- Cytotoxics

Neurological

- **Raised ICP**
  - Tumour
  - Infection
  - Benign intracranial hypertension
- Labyrinthine disorders
- Migraine
- Motion sickness
- Autonomic neuropathy (gastroparesis)

Psychogenic

- Anorexia nervosa
- Bulimia nervosa

Other

- **MI**
- Severe pain, eg testicular torsion, fractures
- Malignancy
- **Acute angle-closure glaucoma**
- Severe coughing, eg chronic bronchitis

> Investigations

Blood tests

- Haematology – FBC, ESR
  - Anaemia (anaemia of chronic disease, malignancy, anorexia)
  - Raised WCC (infection, inflammation)
  - ESR (inflammation, tumour)
- Biochemistry
  - U+Es (dehydration, renal failure, Addison's)
  - Calcium ($\uparrow Ca^{2+} \rightarrow$ vomiting), magnesium (vomiting $\rightarrow$ low Mg^{2+})
  - Glucose (DM, Addison's)
  - CRP (infection)
  - LFTs (cholecystitis, alcohol abuse)
  - Amylase (pancreatitis)
  - Cardiac enzymes – troponin I/T (MI)

Microbiology

- Blood cultures (infection)
- Stool cultures (gastroenteritis)

ECG

- MI

Arterial blood gases

- DKA

Urinalysis

- High specific gravity (dehydration)
- Glucose, ketones (DM)
- Blood (renal colic)
- Blood, WCC, protein (UTI)
- β-hCG (pregnancy test)

Radiology

- CXR
  - Hiatus hernia
  - Aspiration
  - Consolidation
  - Malignancy
- AXR
  - Bowel obstruction
  - Urinary tract calculi
  - Calcified pancreas
  - Faecal loading
- Barium swallow/meal
  - Benign/malignant stricture
  - Pyloric stenosis/gastric outflow obstruction
  - Gastroparesis
- USS
  - Gallstones
- CT head/lumbar puncture
  - Raised ICP
- CT abdomen
  - Staging for intra-abdominal malignancy

OGD ± biopsy and *Helicobacter pylori* status

- Oesophagitis
- Hiatus hernia
- Peptic ulcer
- Carcinoma

Tonometry

- Glaucoma

Further investigations

- 24-hour oesophageal pH studies (GORD)
- Toxicology screen
- Small-bowel contrast study (Crohn's)
- Audiometry (Ménière's disease, labyrinthitis)

Vomiting

Weight loss

➤ History of presenting complaint

Onset

How much weight have you lost and over how long?

Was it intentional, eg dieting, exercise, laxatives/diuretics?

Are there any objective measures of weight loss? (Such as clinical recordings, patient measurements)

Has there been loosening of clothes/tightening of belts? Have you, or others (friends/family), noticed the change? What do you think about it?

Associated symptoms

Is your appetite normal or reduced?

Do you have any dysphagia or pain?

Has there been a change in physical activity?

Precipitating factors

Is your diet adequate? (Poverty, alcohol excess) Has your diet changed recently? Why? *Take a dietary history.*

Are there any symptoms suggestive of malabsorption? (Diarrhoea, abdominal pain, vomiting, steatorrhoea)

Are there any symptoms suggestive of diabetes mellitus? (Polydipsia, polyuria, fatigue, infections)

Are there any symptoms suggestive of hyperthyroidism? (Anxiety, palpitations, tremor, heat intolerance, increased appetite, eye symptoms)

Are there any symptoms suggestive of Addison's disease? (Weakness, dizziness, excessive sweating, skin pigmentation in palmar creases/buccal mucosa/scars/over belt markings)

Are there any biological symptoms of depression? (Lowered mood, reduced appetite, early-morning awakening, suicidal ideation, etc)

Are there any symptoms suggestive of malignancy? (Change in bowel habit, cough, haemoptysis) *Or of chronic infections, such as TB, HIV?* (Fever, malaise, rigors, night sweats, sputum, rashes, lumps and bumps)

Are there any symptoms suggesting major organ dysfunction? (Heart – fatigue, breathlessness, ankle swelling; liver failure; renal failure) *Are there any other cardiac or respiratory symptoms?*

Do you regard your weight as abnormal? Do you think you look thin or normal?

What do you think is wrong?

Ask about treatment already received.

➤ Past medical history

Have you had any serious illnesses in the past?

Is there a history of previous malignancy, thyroid disease, anorexia nervosa, malabsorption, depression or anxiety?

➤ Drug history

Do you take any tablets or injections, such as diuretics, laxatives, diet pills or slimming agents? (Amphetamines)

Compliance, side-effect(s) of medication, OTC/herbal remedies, allergies. (What happens?)

➤ Social history

Do you smoke? How much and for how long have you been smoking? (Smoking reduces appetite)

Do you drink alcohol? (Malnutrition is common in chronic alcoholism)

Have you been abroad? (Overseas travel history, tropical illnesses)

Has there been any contact with infected people?

Recent job changes/loss, separation from partner, depression?

What is your occupation (and its exposures), exercise capacity, lifestyle limitations due to disease?

How far can you usually walk and what stops you?

How do the symptoms interfere with your sleep?

➤ Differential diagnosis

Normal/increased appetite

- Increased demands
  - Growth
  - Malnutrition/neglect
  - Dieting
  - Increase in physical activity
- Diminished absorption
  - Malabsorption (eg **coeliac disease**)
  - Protein-losing enteropathies
  - **Crohn's disease**
  - Drugs
    - ➤ Laxatives
- Increased utilisation
  - **Thyrotoxicosis**
  - Chronic infections (eg pulmonary **TB**)
  - Drugs
    - ➤ Thyroxine
    - ➤ Amphetamine
  - Phaeochromocytoma
  - Anxiety states
- Abnormal calorie loss
  - **Uncontrolled diabetes mellitus**
  - Fistulae
  - Intestinal parasites

Reduced appetite

- Gastrointestinal
  - Dysphagia/odynophagia
  - Peptic ulcer
- Carcinomatosis

- Organ failure
  - Heart (cardiac cachexia)
  - Renal
  - Liver
  - Lung
- Systemic infection
  - Gastroenteritis
  - **HIV/AIDS**
  - **TB**
  - Infective endocarditis
  - Brucellosis
- Systemic inflammation
  - SLE
  - RA
  - Vasculitis
  - Systemic sclerosis
- Endocrine
  - **Addison's disease**
- Drugs
  - Antidepressants
  - L-dopa
  - Digoxin
  - Metformin
  - NSAIDs
  - Opiates
  - Alcohol
  - Heavy smoking
- Psychiatric
  - **Depression**
  - Dementia (senile cachexia)
  - Anorexia nervosa

Weight loss

➤ Investigations

Blood tests

- Haematology – FBC, haematinics, ESR
  - Anaemia (anaemia of chronic disease, malabsorption, renal failure, liver failure)
  - Raised WCC (infection)
  - Serum iron/TIBC/ferritin/vitamin B_{12}/folate
  - ESR (infection, inflammation, malignancy)
- Biochemistry
  - U+Es (renal failure, dehydration, Addison's disease)
  - Ca^{2+} (malnutrition, malignancy)
  - Glucose (insulin-dependent DM)
  - TFTs (hyperthyroidism)
  - CRP (infection)
  - LFTs (liver failure, alcoholism)
  - Albumin (protein-losing enteropathy, malnutrition)
  - HbA_{1c} (diabetic control)
- Immunology
  - Vasculitic/autoimmune screen
  - Antiendomysial, antigliadin, antireticulin, anti-tissue transglutaminase antibodies (coeliac screen)
  - Tumour markers (CEA, CA 125, CA 19-9, α-fetoprotein)
  - HIV serology

Microbiology

- Blood cultures (infection, infective endocarditis)
- Stool
  - M,C+S (gastroenteritis)
  - Faecal fat analysis (malabsoption)
  - Faecal occult blood (colorectal carcinoma)
- TB screen (Mantoux/Heaf test, CXR, sputum/blood M,C+S for AAFBs, bronchoalveolar lavage, pleural aspirate (if effusion), gastric washings, three consecutive early-morning MSUs, needle aspiration, biopsies and histology, X-ray changes of Pott's disease, CSF in TB meningitis, etc)

ECG

- Congestive heart failure

Echocardiography

- Ventricular impairment with CCF

Urinalysis

- Glucose, ketones (DM)
- Proteinuria, blood (renal failure)
- 24-hour collection for urinary metanephrines (phaeochromocytoma)

Radiology

- CXR
  - Carcinoma
  - TB
  - CCF
  - Lymphadenopathy
- AXR
  - Pancreatic calcification with chronic pancreatitis
- USS abdomen
  - Malignancy
  - Small kidneys with chronic renal failure

Further investigations

- OGD ± biopsy (peptic ulcer, carcinoma, coeliac disease)
- Small-bowel enema/follow-through (Crohn's)
- Barium enema (bowel carcinoma)
- Colonoscopy (IBD, bowel carcinoma)
- Short synacthen test (Addison's disease)

Asking difficult questions

This chapter brings together those questions scattered throughout the book that students and doctors find most difficult to ask. Do not attempt to rush into asking these questions – they are difficult to ask and therefore often require a lead statement to prepare the patient for what you are about to ask next. Do not forget that both verbal and non-verbal cues are required to win over the patient's trust in you. You should allow the patient more time to express their feelings and concerns to you.

➤ Sexual history

I need to ask you some important, but rather personal and intimate questions, if I may, which may relate to the symptoms you have been having. Is this okay with you?

Are you currently sexually active?

Do you have a regular partner? For how long?

Have you slept with anyone else recently?

How many partners have you slept with recently?

(For men) Have you ever had sex with another man? (For women) Have you ever had sex with a man known to be bisexual?

Have any of your partners been from another country, or were there any instances while you were abroad?

Do you use barrier contraceptives at all times? Which contraceptive?

Have you had unprotected sex recently?

Have you participated in any risky practices or behaviours recently?

Is/are your partner(s) well?

Have you ever slept with someone who has injected drugs?

Have you noticed any vaginal discharge/discharge from your penis?

Do you experience any pain/discomfort on intercourse?

Asking about erectile dysfunction

Some people with .... (eg diabetes) .... find it difficult to generate or maintain an erection. Do you ever find that this is a problem for you?

Do you find it difficult to relax during intercourse?

I'm sorry I had to ask these questions. I have to ask them routinely of any person who presents with symptoms such as yours. I hope I haven't offended or alarmed you in any way.

➤ Drug abuse

Do you or have you ever used street drugs or recreational drugs of any kind?

Which drugs? How do you take it/them?

How often do you take it/them?

How much do you spend?

Do you, or have you ever injected drugs?

Do you provide your own needles, or have you ever shared needles with other individuals?

➤ Bereavement

I hope you don't mind me asking you this, but has anyone close to you ever died?

Are your parents alive and well?

... I am sorry to hear that. How old were they when they died? May I ask what they died of?

➤ Miscarriages and terminations

I need to ask you some important, but rather personal questions, if I may, as they may relate to the symptoms you have been having. You may, however, find such questions distressing. Is this okay with you? Let me know if you no longer wish to continue.

Have you ever been pregnant before?

Have you ever lost a baby before?

How many times has this happened to you?

At what stage in pregnancy were you on each occasion?

Have you ever had a pregnancy terminated before? Do you mind me asking why? How?

> If you are involved in miscarriage counselling, useful phrases would include:
>
> 'Something goes wrong with the way in which the baby forms from the early stages just after fertilisation.'
>
> 'The problem can be considered as nature's way of preventing an abnormal baby from continuing to grow.'

It is important to stress that it is an event that is beyond the control of the woman herself and unlikely to be influenced by anything that she did or did not do, or any medications or drugs that she did or did not take. This is important to try to lessen the element of guilt or blame, which women may feel.

➤ Infectious contacts

Has anyone close to you been ill recently?

Have you recently come into contact with anyone who has TB/HIV/food poisoning, etc?

➤ Hallucinations and delusions

Do you ever see things or hear noises/voices when there is no one else about?

Have you had any experiences recently that you've found difficult to explain? For example, some people tell me they hear voices when there is no one else around. Does that ever happen to you?

Does your imagination ever play tricks on you?

Do you ever believe you have any special powers?

Have you felt particularly concerned about your safety recently? Why?

Do you ever get the feeling people are talking about you?

Have you felt lately that people are talking about you, plotting about you, or trying to hurt you?

Does anything on TV/radio or in the newspapers have any special meaning for you?

Has it ever appeared that any outside person is interfering with your thoughts in any way?

Do they put in or take away your thoughts?

Do you ever feel other people can hear your thoughts?

Do you ever feel a person outside or an outside force is controlling your actions or feelings?

➤ Suicide/deliberate self-harm

Have things ever got so bad that you have thought about harming yourself or others?

Have you ever felt like giving up, or that your life is not worth living?

Do worrying thoughts ever go through your mind?

Have you ever acted on such thoughts? (Deliberate self-harm or suicide)

How often do these thoughts occur?

Have these thoughts ever included harming someone else as well as yourself?

➤ Urinary/faecal incontinence

Do you ever lose control over your bladder or bowels?

For example, did you lose control over your bladder or bowels during the blackout?

➤ Non-compliance/non-adherence to drug therapy

I realise a lot of people don't take all their tablets. Do you have any problems?

Case scenarios

➤ Case 1

You are the surgical SHO on call. It is midnight. You have accepted a referral from a GP for a 35-year-old woman who has pain in the right iliac fossa.

Please take a detailed history from her to determine the cause of her problem.

What questions would you like to ask the patient?

P C

When you ask the patient what is wrong, she explains that she has had right iliac fossa pain since lunchtime that day. She was out at a restaurant with her best friend and just as she got up from her chair at lunch the pain came on. But she tells you nothing much else until direct questions are asked.

H PC

ODQ the pain came on suddenly.

ODQ the pain has been constant and severe.

ODQ about radiation – The location of the pain is vague and she is unsure whether the pain initially started around the umbilicus but she thinks it may well have. There is no radiation down to the groin. However, ODQ about shoulder-tip pain she agrees that there is radiation to the right shoulder, although she puts this down to a recent shoulder injury that she sustained while playing netball.

ODQ there is no history of trauma to the abdomen.

Associated symptoms:

- Bit of nausea, no vomiting
- No fever
- No distension
- Loss of appetite
- No urinary symptoms (dysuria, urgency, frequency)

- ODQ she has noticed she has passed some vaginal discharge which is dark red and possibly blood but she suspects this is a withdrawal bleed/breakthrough bleeding from the OCP.

Exacerbating factors – Walking around makes the pain worse.

Relieving factors – Lying/sitting still relieves it.

She took ibuprofen earlier but that has not helped.

Severity – The worst pain she has ever had, 9/10. She could never sleep with this pain.

ODQ about her LMP, her last withdrawal bleed (from being on the OCP) was 6 weeks ago.

PMHx

Nil. Has not had her appendix out. No past operations.

No gynaecological history apart from suffering from painful heavy periods as a teenager.

DHx

OCP – No allergies.

ODQ about compliance, she admits that a few weeks ago while on holiday and because of the excitement of being away from home she forgot to take her pill for two consecutive days.

SHx

Functionally independent. Has no children. Shares a flat with a woman friend.

ODQ about travel she recently went on holiday to Ibiza with six other friends, including her boyfriend.

ODQ – Nothing significant about her holiday but she did have a D+V illness from sampling the local delicacies.

Smokes 10 a day and has done since the age of 15.

Drinks about 10 units alcohol a week (ODQ five large glasses of wine a week on average).

ODQ sexual history – She has been going out with her boyfriend for 3 years now. No other sexual partners. ODQ no 'one night stands' on holiday in Ibiza.

FHx

Grandmother diagnosed with bowel cancer at age of 80. Grandfather died of MI at age of 72.

Mother diabetic (insulin-controlled). Father alive and well.

One brother and one sister, alive and well.

SE

Nil. No weight loss.

What is your differential diagnosis?

What investigations would you like to carry out?

Case discussion

This case illustrates well the importance of taking a structured and accurate history in any patient presenting with acute abdominal pain. In this case it would be easy to assume, early on, that the diagnosis is acute appendicitis.

However, further questioning revealed that the patient forgot to take her pill while on holiday in Ibiza with her friends (who included her boyfriend). This, together with the fact that she has also noticed some dark-red vaginal discharge and her last withdrawal bleed is late, puts a **ruptured ectopic pregnancy** at the top of the differential diagnosis. The inefficacy of the OCP due to patient non-compliance was compounded further by a D+V illness while on holiday, which reduces absorption of the drug.

Other diagnoses that would also feature in the differential diagnosis are PID, an ovarian accident (rupture, torsion, haemorrhage), appendicitis, miscarriage, Crohn's disease, etc. However, these are all less likely and this case is an ectopic pregnancy until proved otherwise because of its severity and the consequences of missing such a diagnosis.

This young lady indeed turned out to have an ectopic pregnancy which had ruptured into the peritoneal cavity. Blood within the peritoneal cavity results in chemical peritonitis and irritates the diaphragm, causing referred pain to the shoulder (because the diaphragm is innervated by C3–5). An ectopic pregnancy was confirmed from a positive β-hCG urine test and by transvaginal USS which showed an anembryonic uterus and blood in the cul-de-sac (but no adnexal mass). At laparoscopy she was found to have a ruptured ectopic pregnancy within the right fallopian tube. This was surgically managed and she subsequently made a full recovery.

This case illustrates well the fundamental point of never forgetting to take a full gynaecological history for all women presenting with either acute abdominal pain, amenorrhoea and/or vaginal bleeding. For all women of child-bearing age presenting with such symptoms, always think at the back of your mind – Could this lady be pregnant and now be presenting with a complication of pregnancy?

➤ Case 2

You are the GP of a 39-year-old postman who comes to your practice complaining of a painful red eye.

Please take a history from him to try and determine what is wrong.

What questions would you like to ask the patient?

PC

When you ask the patient what the trouble has been he explains that he has had a three-day history of a painful, left eye.

HPC

Site – Is is truly unilateral and has not had any problems with the contralateral (right) eye.

Onset – It came on quite acutely over a day or so. ODQ no history trauma/foreign bodies to eye.

Character – ODQ it is actual pain rather than discomfort/irritation/itching/dryness or a gritty eye. No obvious diurnal variation in symptoms.

Radiation – No headache, no radiation.

Associated symptoms:
- ODQ he has noticed vision has become more blurred in that eye when he covers up the other eye.
- ODQ no changes to colour vision.
- ODQ parts of the visual field are not obviously missing.
- ODQ no eye discharge or stickiness.
- ODQ no nausea/vomiting.
- ODQ eye has been watering.
- ODQ no rhinorrhoea.

Timing – It has been getting worse over the past few days.

Exacerbating factors – Light (photophobia).

No **R**elieving factors.

Severity – Pain 8–9/10. He normally wears disposable contact lenses but has been unable to do so over the last few days because the pain is so bad.

ODQ the patient also has noticed that over the past six months, or so, he has had generalised aches and pains in his joints but particularly his lower back. He attributes this to his job.

ODQ he describes a bit of loose stools (on and off for the last few months), ODQ with slime and mucus but no blood. No fever. ODQ mild abdominal tenderness but nothing compared to his eye pain.

ODQ no urethral discharge. No other urogenital symptoms.

No contacts with a similar problem. No SOB or skin changes.

PMHx

ODQ no history of glaucoma.

No history of previous eye problems. Contact lens hygiene is good.

Only history of note is a meniscal tear ten years previously sustained whilst playing football.

ODQ no history of headaches or migraines. ODQ no history of psoriasis. ODQ no history of ankylosing spondylitis.

DHx

- Paracetamol for pain.
- NKDA

SHx

Smokes 10 a day for 20 years. Drinks 15 units alcohol a week.

Lives with his girlfriend. Functionally independent.

ODQ no new sexual partners recently.

ODQ not IVDU.

FHx

Nil. ODQ he thinks his grandfather (maternal side) had glaucoma.

SE

Nil. No weight change.

What is your differential diagnosis?

What investigations would you like to carry out?

Case discussion

The history is fairly vague but indicates favourably a diagnosis of an **acute iritis** (anterior uveitis). The features that fit with this are a unilateral, painful, watering red eye of relatively acute onset, that is exacerbated by light and is associated with a loss of visual acuity.

Having said that, the diagnosis of an **acute angle-closure glaucoma** presenting in this way should **always** be at the back of one's mind and can present in a similar fashion, although there are no systemic symptoms here (such as nausea and vomiting) which usually accompanies acute angle-closure glaucoma. The pre-test probability of glaucoma is increased further in this case by the presence of a positive family history. Tonometry should be a mandatory part of the examination in **all** such cases where a patient presents with a unilateral painful red eye and should never be forgotten as the condition is potentially sight-threatening. **Never forget that missing a diagnosis of acute angle-closure glaucoma may result in permanent visual loss.**

The other differential that should also feature high up in the differential diagnosis is an infectious process in view of the fact that the patient is normally a contact lenses wearer, although he wears disposable lenses and hygiene is good so this makes an infection due to contact lenses less likely. However, it does not rule out the possibility of an inflammatory process within the cornea (keratitis, corneal abrasion, corneal ulceration, dendritic ulcer etc.).

Having considered the possibility that this may be an iritis the astute clinician should try to find out the possible cause for such a process. The fact that ODQ the patient describes what sounds like sacro-iliitis makes the possibility of an **HLA-B27 associated disease** more likely for the cause for his iritis. There is no history of psoriasis or ankylosing spondylitis, or nothing from the sexual history to indicate a possible Reiter's syndrome (no urethral discharge). In view of the loose stools and associated mucus this makes the possibility of an enteropathic arthritis associated with inflammatory bowel disease, or a reactive arthritis associated with infective diarrhoea, more likely. Indeed this patient turned out to be within the 10% of patients with inflammatory bowel disease that initially present with extra-intestinal manifestations of the disease as their main presenting problem (in this case an acutely painful red eye as an extra-intestinal manifestation of ulcerative colitis).

➤ Case 3

You are the resident medical house officer on call. You accept the referral from a GP for a 73-year-old lady who collapsed earlier that day and had what the GP thinks was a seizure.

When you arrive at the bedside the patient is alert and orientated and is accompanied by her daughter who witnessed the whole episode.

What questions would you like to ask the patient?

PC

When you ask them what happened they explain that they were out shopping together at the supermarket when suddenly her eyes rolled back and she collapsed to the ground and started fitting.

HPC

➤ Pre-episode

ODQ the patient doesn't remember what happened and thinks she may have blacked out for a few seconds (ie there was probable LOC). ODQ about a warning the patient explains that there was no clear warning. ODQ no chest pain, chest tightness or breathlessness or palpitations. ODQ about the colour of patient's face the daughter explains that she went very grey and looked dead. ODQ about posture, the patient had been leaning on the trolley (because her walking is not that good) and then stood up just prior to the episode. ODQ no sweatiness/clamminess prior to the fall.

➤ During episode

ODQ there was erratic movement of the limbs. The episode lasted seconds rather than minutes but the daughter says it felt like longer. ODQ no tongue biting, urinary/faecal incontinence. ODQ breathing was laboured during the episode. ODQ the patient hit her head when she fell to the ground and bruised the left side of her face. The daughter did not take her pulse during the episode.

➤ *Post-episode*

ODQ the patient made a rapid recovery over seconds. ODQ there was no real weakness apart from aches and pain on the areas which she fell on. ODQ she doesn't remember too much about the episode. ODQ about the colour of her face, colour returned rapidly to her face after the episode. ODQ she remained on the floor, supine, until the paramedics arrived and brought her to hospital.

ODQ she has never had an episode like this before.

ODQ about each of the cardiovascular risk factors:

- No cardiac history
- Ex-smoker (15/day for 30 years but gave up at the age of 50)
- Not known to have high cholesterol
- Hypertensive (ODQ for 15 years)
- Diabetic (ODQ insulin-controlled for 40 years)
- Positive family history (father died of MI at age of 46)

PMHx

Type 1 DM for 40 years. Insulin-controlled.

Hypertension for 15 years.

Gout.

DHx

- 2.5 mg bendroflumethiazide once daily PO
- 50 mg atenolol once daily PO
- Mixtard 30 insulin
- Allopurinol
- No known drug allergies

SHx

ODQ lives alone.

ODQ has carers that come in twice weekly to help with the cleaning and cooking.

ODQ daughter lives 5 minutes' drive away and visits daily and assists with shopping.

ODQ walks with a stick with a normal exercise tolerance of around 100 yards on flat.

Ex-smoker (15 a day for 30 years).

Alcohol negligible.

FHx

Father died of MI at 46.

Sister had epilepsy.

What is your differential diagnosis?

What investigations would you like to carry out?

Case discussion

This case illustrates well the importance of taking a thorough history from any patient with collapse 'query cause' in whom the differential is large and when individual diagnoses are sometimes hard to tease apart. However, as usual, the history gives a substantial clue as to the cause. This case is not so easy – there are many different traps to fall into here and the potential causes for this lady's collapse are varied.

The brief LOC precipitated by a change in posture (from leaning on a trolley to the standing position) makes one think of **orthostatic hypotension**, especially in view of the fact that the patient is on multiple antihypertensive treatments. However, what counts against this argument is that there was no clear warning or dizziness prior to the event, which one would expect with orthostatic hypotension. That the patient sustained an injury to her face from the collapse is testament to the fact that there was no clear warning to allow protective mechanisms (ie an outstretched hand) to set in to prevent injury to the face. This suggests a cause more sinister than orthostatic hypotension for her collapse. Having said that, a **diabetic autonomic neuropathy** in an elderly patient is still on the cards with this history.

Yet another potential cause for this woman's collapse is **hypoglycaemia**. The logic behind this is that she said that she was a type 1 diabetic, controlled on insulin. It is perfectly feasible that she may have taken too much insulin that morning by mistake or took the usual dose of insulin but has not eaten enough, precipitating a hypoglycaemic episode. The fact that she is on a β-blocker means that the usual warning symptoms of a hypoglycaemic episode, such as palpitations, would be masked. If this were a hypoglycaemic episode, however, the patient may have noticed clamminess/sweating prior to the fall or neuroglycopenic symptoms such as confusion, drowsiness, etc. Nonetheless, this was not the case.

It is perfectly reasonable to include a diagnosis of an **epileptiform seizure** (not strictly epilepsy as this is a first seizure) in the differential diagnosis on the basis of the history. What counts against this is that there was no tongue biting/incontinence, movement of the limbs was erratic rather than symmetrical and rhythmical, the duration of the episode was in seconds rather than in minutes and the usual post-ictal features that one would expect were not present (ie there was no evidence of Todd's paresis and there was no post-ictal confusion/headache/aches and pains/ feeling of being washed out, etc).

The diagnosis that must be entertained and is most likely on the basis of the history is a cardiac event. This is an elderly patient with clearly significant cardiovascular risk factors and a positive family history for cardiovascular disease. The fact there was no clear warning for the event, along with a rapid recovery, and coupled with the daughter's description of a look of greyness about her mother prior to the fall argues in favour of a diagnosis of **cardiac syncope** or a **Stokes–Adams episode**. Although there was no chest pain or tightness prior to the event, this is not mandatory to make such a diagnosis, especially in an elderly, diabetic patient like this one. This is because a significant proportion of these patients will have a 'silent' cardiac event with no chest pain whatsoever, as a result of associated autonomic neuropathy. The convulsions again can be a manifestation of cardiac syncope and are due to brain hypoxia, resulting from reduced cardiac output associated with the cardiac event. However, the other possibility that must be entertained is that when she hit her head on the way down, the injury sustained might have resulted in an intracerebral bleed that could have induced a seizure. Hence the requirement for a CT head to exclude the possibility of a haematoma.

This patient ended up with a 24-hour tape which showed episodes of third-degree atrioventricular block. She was listed for a permanent pacemaker and following this had no further episodes of collapse.

> Case 4

You are a GP. A 63-year-old female teacher presents to your practice with weight loss.

Please take a full history from the patient to determine the cause.

What questions would you like to ask the patient?

PC

When you ask the patient what is wrong she explains that she is concerned that she is losing weight based on her own view of herself and what others around her have noticed.

HPC

ODQ she explains that she is normally 11 stone.

ODQ she has lost around 2 stone in weight.

ODQ over 3 months.

ODQ her appetite is unchanged and normal for her.

ODQ about associated symptoms she explains that she is more tired than usual and her ankles are more swollen than usual. She has hip pain from a recent fractured neck of femur on the right.

ODQ no PR bleeding, haematemesis, dysphagia, breathlessness, chest pain, haematuria, jaundice, haemoptysis, breast lumps.

ODQ about a change in bowel habit the patient describes a change in stool frequency.

ODQ she is passing stool more often than usual (2–3 x daily instead of the usual once).

ODQ her stools are darker than normal (ever since starting the iron tablets).

ODQ (now you mention it) her stools do float in the pan and are more difficult to flush away than usual.

ODQ no palpitations, heat intolerance, neck lumps, eye changes, tremor, skin changes.

ODQ sometimes gets dizzy upon standing.

ODQ no polyuria or polydipsia.

PMHx

Hypothyroidism

Unexplained iron deficiency anaemia – she is awaiting an OGD and barium enema

Mild congestive heart failure with swelling of ankles.

Osteoporosis.

Recent fractured right neck of femur + dynamic hip screw repair (2 months ago).

DHx

- 100 mcg thyroxine OD PO
- 200 mg ferrous sulphate TDS PO
- 40 mg furosemide OD
- 20 mg BD MST for hip pain

ODQ not on HRT.

Allergic to penicillin

SHx

Smokes 10 a day and has been since age 15.

Drinks 20 units/week.

Lives with her husband. Both fit and well.

FHx

None of note. Both parents alive and well. No siblings.

What is your differential diagnosis?

What investigations would you like to carry out?

Case discussion

The most important determinant in taking a history from a patient with weight loss is finding out if it is associated with a reduced, a normal or an increased appetite. Only then can the various causes of weight loss be distinguished effectively in the history.

For example, although the patient suffers with mild **congestive cardiac failure** and has noticed increased ankle swelling, the fact that the loss in weight is associated with a normal appetite, rather than a reduced appetite, suggests that this is not the sole cause for her weight loss, especially a 2 stone loss in weight in the last 3 months.

The patient is noted to be normally **hypothyroid** and is on thyroxine replacement treatment. Thus if the patient is taking too high a maintenance dose of thyroxine than is actually required then she will become thyrotoxic and lose weight. However, again this possibility is less likely in view of the normal, rather than increased appetite and the lack of thyrotoxic symptoms, such as tremor, palpitations etc.

An important cause for weight loss that should always be considered is **Addison's disease** which often presents very non-specifically. Indeed, the most reliable and sensitive initial presenting feature of Addison's disease is weight loss. This diagnosis is supported by the patient reporting episodes of dizzy spells upon assuming the upright position, although this may be related more to the furosemide she is taking causing orthostatic hypotension. Another feature which makes the diagnosis more likely is the associated hypothyroidism which we can assume is probably autoimmune in nature and may be associated with Addison's disease. However, against a diagnosis of Addison's disease is the fact that the patient's appetite is not markedly reduced and there are no reported skin changes (although this may be subtle). Nevertheless, this would be an important diagnosis to exclude.

In a lady of this age group one must always consider a diagnosis of **malignancy** as a cause of weight loss and this would feature high up in the differential diagnosis as cancer, unlike Addison's disease, is common. The patient has an unexplained iron deficiency anaemia and has sustained a possible pathological fracture. Both these features make a diagnosis of malignancy even more likely. The patient has not noticed any PR bleeding although her stools are darker then normal but this may be attributed to the iron tablets. Malignancy must be excluded and the GP was right to organise an OGD/barium enema to exclude a gastrointestinal malignancy, in view of the iron deficiency anaemia and the reported change in bowel habit. Other potential sources of malignancy in this case are multiple myeloma, and carcinoma of the breast, lung, kidney and thyroid.

However, what the astute clinician would have picked up on is weight loss in the face of a normal appetite and steatorrhoea (ie increased stool bulk/frequency associated with pale (putty coloured), offensive stools that float in the pan and are difficult to flush away), although her stools were not strictly pale in this case because she is taking iron sulphate tablets. In view of weight loss and steatorrhoea and the fact that the patient has an unexplained iron deficiency anaemia, a diagnosis of **coeliac disease** (or gluten-sensitive enteropathy) must be entertained, which can indeed present for the first time in someone of this age group. The associated malabsorption from coeliac disease can lead to an iron deficiency anaemia and a hypoalbuminaemic state (hence the reported increased ankle swelling). Such patients are also at an increased risk of osteoporosis as a result of calcium and vitamin D malabsorption. This can lead to an increased fracture risk, as in this case, especially as the patient was not on bone prophylaxis or HRT.

The GP requested a coeliac screen and she was found to be positive for anti-tissue transglutaminase antibodies. A small bowel biopsy confirmed the diagnosis. The patient was commenced on a gluten free diet and she regained weight rapidly. The swelling of ankles and iron deficiency anaemia gradually resolved with time.

➤ Case 5

A 62-year-old female judge has been referred by her GP to your neurology clinic with a principal complaint of headaches.

Please take a history from her and come to an appropriate diagnosis.

What questions would you like to ask the patient?

PC

When you ask the patient about her problem she explains that she suffers with headaches. Her GP is unsure as to the exact cause for them so he has referred her to you for a specialist opinion.

HPC

ODQ she has had the headaches for the past 6 weeks.

ODQ she was well before this and has never suffered with headaches like this.

Site – ODQ the headaches are bilateral and frontal.

Onset – ODQ the headaches are present all the time. They were gradual in onset.

Character – ODQ the pain is a dull ache/nagging pain.

Radiation – ODQ none.

Associated symptoms:

- ODQ no aura/changes in vision/fortification spectra/zigzags/ scintillating scotomas
- ODQ no weakness/changes in speech/fits/changes in personality
- ODQ no fever/neck stiffness/photophobia
- ODQ no nausea or vomiting
- ODQ no red eye/rhinorrhoea/nasal disturbances
- ODQ no galactorrhoea
- ODQ malaise, generalised aches and pains
- ODQ low mood
- ODQ mild weight loss (few pounds over last 6 weeks)

Timing – Getting worse.

ODQ about diurnal variation, she explains that it is present throughout the day but slightly worse in the evenings and at weekends.

Exacerbating/relieving factors:

- ODQ nothing especially makes it better or worse.
- ODQ not exacerbated by coughing or straining.
- However, on ODQ about pain on chewing food or cleaning her teeth she explains that this aggravates the pain.
- In addition, ODQ about combing her hair she explains that this also aggravates the pain.

Severity – The worst headaches she has ever experienced, 9/10. Keeps her awake at night. ODQ has affected her work which is bothering her a great deal.

PMHx

ODQ not previously a migraine sufferer.

ODQ does not suffer from glaucoma.

Nil significant PMHx, except a cholecystectomy in 2002 for biliary colic.

ODQ no previous head injuries.

DHx

- Hormone replacement therapy
- Amitriptyline 25 mg nocte PO
- Paracetamol PRN PO

SHx

High-powered and stressful job.

Married with four children who are grown-up and have all left home.

The last child left home when the headaches started 6 weeks ago.

ODQ currently experiencing marriage difficulties.

Non-smoker.

On average, four small glasses of red wine per week. No spirits.

FHx

Nil significant.

What is your differential diagnosis?

What investigations would you like to carry out?

Case discussion

Headaches are common in general practice and this means the history is imperative if serious causes are to be effectively identified and treated.

At first glance this seems to be a simple case of **tension headache**, especially as the headache is bilateral, frontal, gnawing and constant in nature and is associated with various stressful life events (job, marriage difficulties, kids leaving home, not sleeping, etc). **Migraine** is another possible diagnosis, although there is no aura associated with it which would make this common migraine rather then the variety associated with aura (classic migraine). However, there are no features here to suggest a typical migraine – there are no systemic symptoms such as nausea or vomiting, the headache is constant rather than intermittent and the patient does not describe feeling washed out afterwards, or wishing to sleep or spend time in a dark room, which migraineurs often report.

Analgesia rebound headaches are a possibility and can feature as a cause of headache in patients like this. However, again, the nature of the headache, the severity, and that it is constant rather than intermittent argue in favour of something more sinister.

The diagnosis is given away by a positive finding of jaw claudication (pain on eating and teeth brushing) and scalp tenderness (pain on combing her hair), as well as the accompanying symptoms of malaise, weight loss and generalised aches and pains (associated PMR).

The diagnosis is indeed **giant cell (temporal) arteritis**. She is unable to sleep at night because the pain is so bad. That the headache is worse in the evening can probably be attributed to the pain being exacerbated by resting her head on a pillow at night which elicits scalp tenderness. Such a diagnosis should never be forgotten in any patient over the age of 50 as, if missed, it can result in irreversible blindness as a result of anterior ischaemic optic neuropathy.

The ESR came back at 142 mm/h. She was commenced on steroids and bone prophylaxis immediately and, with time, the ESR gradually returned to normal. A temporal artery biopsy confirmed the diagnosis.

➤ Case 6

You are a GP. A 30-year-old man comes to your practice complaining of a neck lump.

Please take a full history from the patient in order to try and determine what is wrong.

What questions would you like to ask the patient?

P C

When you ask the patient what has been the trouble he explains that he has been troubled by a lump in his neck which is getting larger with time.

H PC

ODQ duration for 3 weeks.

Site – ODQ confined to neck. ODQ multiple lumps rather than a single lump.

Onset – Lump came up over a day or two.

Character – Smooth, fairly soft. ODQ non-tender lumps.

Associated symptoms:

- ODQ no fever, no weight change.
- ODQ malaise.
- ODQ no scrotal or other swellings.
- ODQ pruritus.
- ODQ pruritus which is generalised, rather than localised, and is especially bad at night.
- ODQ night sweats.
- ODQ no SOB, cough, sputum, haemoptysis, pharyngitis.
- ODQ no change in bowel habit, palpitations, heat/cold intolerance, tremor, voice changes, hair changes.

Timing – Getting worse with time.

Exacerbating/relieving factors – None.

Severity – worried about cosmetic effect and whether others will start noticing it.

PMHx

ODQ no recent cat scratches.

ODQ no recent viral illnesses/pharyngitis.

ODQ has not come in to contact with people with known TB as far as he is aware.

Known epileptic.

DHx

- Phenytoin (ODQ been on for 8 years)
- NKDA

SHx

Car mechanic. Lives with parents.

Smokes 10 a day for 10 years

Drinks 20 units per week

Has experimented with drugs on one occasion 3 months ago. ODQ via intravenous route.

Sexual history – ODQ multiple partners in the last 6 months. ODQ he did have unprotected sex one night 3 months ago with a girl he hardly knew. He does not keep in contact with her and has not seen her since.

No significant travel history.

FHx

Nil

What is your differential diagnosis?

What investigations would you like to carry out?

Case discussion

It is clear from the patient's history that what he is describing is regional lymphadenopathy of the neck lymph nodes. This is favoured by his description of multiple neck lumps.

Having reached this far the next question to ask is what is actually causing this. The causes are numerous but is complicated by the very fact that he is taking **phenytoin** which itself can cause lymphadenopathy. However, in view of the relatively short history of the presenting complaint compared with the duration he has been on phenytoin treatment makes a diagnosis of drug-induced lymphadenopathy less likely.

The diagnostician is left to decipher out the remaining main causes of this gentleman's neck lymphadenopathy, most notably infectious causes (TB, HIV here) and malignant causes.

TB is a possible cause for this gentleman's problem but he does not have any respiratory symptoms and he has not been in contact with anyone with known TB, although he does suffer with night sweats. He is, on the other hand, at high risk of acquiring **HIV** especially in view of his significant past sexual history and the very fact that he has experimented with intravenous drugs. An HIV test (coupled with HIV counselling) in addition to a CXR would be therefore be appropriate investigations to exclude TB and HIV respectively. Other infectious causes (such as EBV, CMV, toxoplasmosis) are possible but less likely on the basis of the history.

The key to this case was picking up on the associated pruritus and night sweats which in association with multiple non-tender lymphadenopathy indicates a diagnosis of **lymphoma**. A diagnosis of nodular sclerosing **Hodgkin's disease** was later confirmed on lymph node biopsy.

➤ Case 7

A 47-year-old lady comes to your GP practice complaining of fatigue.

Please proceed to take a history from her to determine to cause of her lethargy.

What questions would you like to ask the patient?

P C

When you ask her what is wrong she explains that she has been feeling 'run down' for the past couple of weeks. She says it is affecting both her work and her life outside work. She offers no more information in response to the initial open-ended question.

HPC

ODQ she is unclear when it exactly started because it came on gradually but says it has been at least 6–8 weeks.

ODQ she feels subjectively low and tired all the time.

ODQ she has had difficulty sleeping at night but is not troubled by early morning waking.

ODQ this is because she is worried by her recent separation from her husband and she is left to look after her two children on her own.

ODQ she is no longer able to enjoy the things that she used to enjoy doing (ie reading, watching TV, meeting friends). Whether this is because of marriage difficulties she is unsure.

ODQ she has not thought of harming herself and her suicidal risk is low.

ODQ decreased ability to think or concentrate.

ODQ weight gain (1/2 stone over last 2–3 months). ODQ normal appetite.

ODQ about **each** of the following she has noticed:

- She is mildly more constipated than usual.
- She is experiencing heavier periods than usual.
- She is more sensitive of the cold and has to turn her home heating on even though it is July!
- No voice changes.
- No hair changes.

PMHx

ODQ no history of psychiatric illnesses or depression.

Only past medical history of note is fibroids and asthma.

Pulmonary embolus 5 months ago.

DHx

- Salbutamol inhaler.
- Seretide inhaler.
- Warfarin OD PO (dose as per INR)
- NKDA

SHx

ODQ works as a secretary. No current job problems.

ODQ lives with her 2 children.

ODQ recently separated from her husband (ODQ 1 month ago, shortly after her symptoms started).

Smokes 25 per day for 30 years.

Drinks 30 units alcohol per week (mainly gin).

FHx

Nil

What is your differential diagnosis?

What investigations would you like to carry out?

Case discussion

Initially this lady seems to give a very good history for a **depressive disorder** in view of her biological symptoms of lethargy, difficulty sleeping, weight gain, subjectively low mood, anhedonia and general lack in her ability to concentrate on the things she used to enjoy. This seems to be triggered by a potential exogenous cause, namely her recent separation from her husband and having to take full responsibility for the children alone.

However, the perceptive clinician would have picked up on the fact that her symptoms actually commenced **before** her marriage break-up, although she was probably having marriage difficulties prior to the actual separation. What really gives the diagnosis away, however, are the organic symptoms she describes of constipation, heavy vaginal bleeding (which may also be related to fibroids or dysfunctional uterine bleeding as a result of her perimenopausal state) and cold intolerance. The diagnosis is of course **hypothyroidism**.

Hypothyroidism is one of the great masqueraders of clinical medicine as it can present in so many different ways and to so many different specialists. It is an important diagnosis not to miss as it is so easily treated and is one of the reversible causes of both depression and dementia.

Her TSH, T4 levels and thyroid autoantibodies were consistent with a diagnosis of autoimmune primary hypothyroidism. She was commenced on thyroxine replacement therapy and her depressive illness, fatigue and other symptoms rapidly resolved. This case serves to illustrate that whenever a patient seems depressed, or presents with features of a psychiatric illness, always think at the back of your mind could an organic disorder better explain this patient's symptomatology. Only consider a psychiatric illness when all possible organic conditions have been effectively excluded.

➤ Case 8

A 62-year-old gentleman is admitted to Accident and Emergency with chest pain.

Please take a history to determine the cause.

What questions would you like to ask the patient?

PC

When you ask the patient what is wrong he explains that he was on the golf course today when he experienced an episode of chest pain. His golfing partner called 999 for an ambulance.

HPC

Site – Central.

Onset – ODQ it came on quite acutely at the tee of the ninth hole. ODQ no history of trauma.

Character – ODQ the patient describes the pain 'like a weight' on his chest, as if someone is sitting on him.

Radiation – ODQ associated back pain.

Associated symptoms – ODQ no palpitations, breathlessness, syncope, sweating, N+V, fever.

ODQ he has noticed his vision has slightly deteriorated following the chest pain.

ODQ he has noticed that his right hand is 'clumsier' since the chest pain commenced.

Timing – The chest pain at its worst lasted approximately 20 minutes but it has been with him the whole time since it began (in total 45 minutes thus far).

Exacerbating factors – Nothing in particular. ODQ the pain is not affected by breathing.

No **R**elieving factors.

Severity – Pain 10/10. The worst pain he has ever experienced.

ODQ about each of the cardiovascular risk factors:

- Not diabetic
- Hypertensive (ODQ for 10 years and poorly controlled)
- Patient unsure about cholesterol status
- Smokes approximately 20 a day (ODQ for 42 years)
- Nil past cardiac history
- Positive family history (brother died of MI at the age of 46)

PMHx

Normally fit and well. No previous illnesses or operations.

ODQ no cardiac history and he has never suffered with angina previously.

DHx

- Atenolol 50 mg once daily PO (for hypertension)
- ODQ never been thrombolysed before
- Allergic to penicillin
- ODQ about adherence to medications, the patient admits that he is not very good at taking his tablets.

SHx

Lives with his wife in a bungalow. Normally functionally independent.

ODQ smokes approximately 20 per day and has done since the ago of 20.

ODQ drinks a couple of pints of beer most evenings.

FHx

Brother died of an MI at the age of 46.

What is your differential diagnosis?

What investigations would you like to carry out?

Case discussion

Chest pain is a common presenting complaint and therefore features commonly both in primary/secondary care settings and in examinations. There are **four causes** of chest pain that demand immediate management – **MI**, **aortic dissection**, **tension pneumothorax** and **PE**. The aim of the chest pain history is therefore to be as thorough and as succinct as possible to identify or exclude any of these four possible causes which require the initiation of immediate management.

In view of the character of the chest pain and the presence of the cardiovascular risk factors, at first glance this chest pain seems to represent an underlying MI. However, the associated visual disturbances and weakness of his right hand should trigger alarm bells in the back of one's mind about the possibility of a CVA, either as a result of an aortic dissection, or as a result of an embolic event caused by mural thrombus formation following a myocardial infarct. Clues supporting the former possibility are the severity of the pain and the associated radiation of the pain to the back.

This indeed turned out to be a case of **aortic dissection**. CXR showed a widened mediastinum. This was followed by a CT chest with contrast where a dissection was noted running from the aortic arch, down the length of the aorta, up to and including the renal arteries. There was also involvement of aortic side branches, including the left common carotid artery (leading to a CVA with visual disturbances and clumsiness of the right hand). A transoesophageal echocardiogram defined the location of the intimal tear and the patient was subsequently managed accordingly.

In summary, never forget the four serious causes of chest pain that necessitate immediate management: acute MI, tension pneumothorax, PE and aortic dissection. In any patient presenting with chest pain, always consider the possibility of an aortic dissection if there are any unusual associated symptoms, or if the history does not fit with a simple case of MI.

➤ Case 9

A 65-year-old lady comes to see you (her GP) complaining of
generalised muscle aches and pains. She is keen to find out what is
wrong.

Please proceed to take a full history from her to try to determine the
cause for her problem.

What questions would you like to ask the patient?

P C

When you enquire into the patient's problem she explains that she has
general muscle aches and pains and that she has been feeling low and
weak for some time.

HPC

Site – All over, but especially the lower back.

Onset – ODQ it came on about 6 weeks ago, about the same time that
she retired from work.

Character – ODQ the patient describes the pain as 'aching'. ODQ no
diurnal variation.

Radiation – ODQ radiates all over.

Associated symptoms – Weakness (ODQ due to pain rather than true
weakness).

ODQ associated weight loss – half a stone over 2 months.

ODQ no fever, visual changes, headache, skin rashes, eye problems.

ODQ no constipation, memory loss, hair changes, voice changes, ankle
swelling, neck lumps.

Timing – The pain is there all the time, including at night.

Exacerbating factors – Nothing in particular.

NSAIDs and a warm bath sometimes help to relieve the pain.

Severity – Pain 8/10. It disrupts sleep and keeps her awake at night.
ODQ on occasions it has woken her up from her sleep.

ODQ about her concerns/ideas/expectations, she believes it may be her
thyroid playing up.

PMHx

ODQ no recent viral illnesses or upper/lower respiratory tract infections.

Hysterectomy 15 years ago.

Hypercholesterolaemia.

DHx

- Simvastatin 40 mg nocte (ODQ on this for 2 years with no previous problems)
- Amitriptyline 25 mg nocte (ODQ on this for 6 weeks)
- Ibuprofen PRN for pain
- No known drug allergies

SHx

Recently retired from teaching.

Divorced, no children.

Non-smoker and never has done.

Negligible alcohol intake.

Feels her life is 'empty' now she has left work.

FHx

Nil.

What is your differential diagnosis?

What investigations would you like to carry out?

Case discussion

The causes of generalised muscle aches and pains are numerous and a careful history will usually permit the practitioner to distinguish the various causes. Although **fibromyalgia** or **chronic fatigue syndrome** or **depression** are possible causes for this woman's problem, especially in the light of the recent stressful life events (divorce, recently retired, life feeling empty), they should remain diagnoses of exclusion, especially as symptoms have only been present for around 6 weeks.

It is theoretically possible that the patient's problem may be caused by **simvastatin** (which can cause a severe, unpredictable drug-induced myositis with rhabdomyolysis in 0.5% of patients). This would be an absolute indication to stop the drug immediately. However, this is less likely as ODQ the patient has been on simvastatin for 2 years, with no prior problems or reactions. It must, however, be kept at the back of one's mind as a potential cause for this patient's symptoms.

A **viral illness** (such as influenza) is possible, although such symptoms should have resolved after about 6 weeks. Viral serology may nonetheless be helpful. **Hypothyroidism** is another possible cause for this lady's presenting complaint, although the absence of organic features of hypothyroidism (such as constipation, memory loss, hair changes, hoarse voice, etc) makes this less likely.

A diagnosis of **PMR**, **inflammatory myopathy** (eg dermatomyositis, polymyositis) or another connective tissue disease would be consistent with this patient's history and should be excluded by ESR and CPK ± autoimmune profile, respectively. A diagnosis of **osteomalacia** is also possible and serum calcium, phosphorus and alkaline phosphatase should also be requested.

However, in view of the patient's age and associated weight loss, a diagnosis of **malignancy** must be entertained (especially **multiple myeloma** which often presents as non-specifically as this). Indeed, this patient was found to have Bence Jones proteinuria, a monoclonal IgG band with immunoparesis on serum electrophoresis, and a skeletal survey revealed multiple lytic lesions throughout the bony skeleton. A bone marrow biopsy confirmed a diagnosis of multiple myeloma.

In summary, never forget **multiple myeloma** as a cause of non-specific aches and pains in middle-aged and elderly patients. In such cases always request a myeloma screen.

➤ Case 10

A 52-year-old gentleman comes to see you with difficulty swallowing.

Please proceed to take a history to determine what is wrong.

What questions would you like to ask the patient?

PC

When you ask the patient what the main problem is he explains that swallowing is becoming increasingly difficult.

HPC

ODQ he has had difficulty swallowing for about 4 weeks.

ODQ no history of foreign body ingestion.

ODQ at present he has difficulty swallowing both solids and liquids. ODQ he initially only had difficulty swallowing solids.

ODQ it is continuous rather than intermittent.

ODQ no drooling of saliva.

ODQ food seems to get stuck at the level of the thyroid cartilage.

ODQ no pain on swallowing (odynophagia).

ODQ associated weight loss – 1 stone over 3 months and ODQ his clothes have got looser.

ODQ no abdominal pain, heartburn/dyspepsia, haematemesis.

ODQ no other muscle weakness elsewhere, or skin changes.

PMHx

RTA at the age of 25.

Nil else.

DHx

- Nil
- No known drug allergies

SHx

Smokes 30 per day and has done since the age of 20.

20 units alcohol per week (two to three glasses of wine per night).

Lives with wife. Has two children.

Normally fit and well.

FHx

Nil significant.

What is your differential diagnosis?

What investigations would you like to carry out?

Case discussion

Dysphagia is disproportionately common in examinations and is a relatively easy history to score highly on if prepared for adequately. The key features to determine early on from the patient is whether the dysphagia is continuous or intermittent (stricture vs neuromuscular cause), whether initially it was to solids, liquids, or both, along with the sequence of events that followed (initially to solids and then progressing to both solids and liquids suggests an oesophageal stricture; initially to liquids suggests a neuromuscular cause). Finally, if a stricture is presumed likely, it is imperative in the history to distinguish a benign (peptic) stricture from a malignant stricture (weight loss, history of dyspepsia/ haematemesis/ PUD, associated abdominal pain, etc).

Thus, in this case, a history of continuous dysphagia, initially to solids and then progressing to both solids and liquids suggests the presence of an **oesophageal stricture**. Coupled with a history of significant weight loss and the absence of features of PUD, this suggests the presence of a **malignant** oesophageal stricture.

An OGD in this man revealed a tight oesophageal stricture 25 cm from the incisors, with a malignant-looking appearance. Biopsies were taken which revealed adenocarcinoma of the oesophagus.

➤ Case 11

You are a GP Foundation Year doctor. A 65-year-old man has come to see you complaining of pink urine.

Please take a detailed history from him to determine the cause of the problem.

What questions would you like to ask the patient?

PC

When you ask the patient what is wrong, he explains that he has noticed pink urine for the last 3 weeks. He tells you nothing much else until direct questions are asked.

HPC

No recent beetroot ingestion.

Onset, nature and character – frank haematuria apparent every time he passes urine and throughout the stream. Never had previous episodes. No clots.

Associated symptoms:

ODQ mild, dull ache around the right loin (constant, does not radiate).

Urinary symptoms – no symptoms of dysuria or prostatism (no hesitancy, poor stream, terminal dribbling, nocturia, incontinence).

Systemic features – no fever or night sweats, there has been some weight loss (half stone over 6 weeks, with belt becoming looser on trousers).

No history of trauma.

PMHx

Past medical history includes paroxysmal AF and hypertension.

Specifically, no history prostate pathology or urinary calculi.

DHx

Amiodarone 200 mg OD and warfarin for AF.

Also takes simvastatin 40 mg nocte and amlodipine 5 md OD

NKDA. No OTC medications.

SHx

Functionally independent.

Smokes 15 a day and has done since the age of 17.

Drinks 24 units alcohol a week.

No recent travel history.

FHx

No FHx of note. Three children well, both parents died in their 80s of cardiovascular disease.

SE

Nil

What is your differential diagnosis?

What investigations would you like to carry out?

Case discussion

Macroscopic haematuria should always be taken seriously and should be regarded as cancerous in origin until proven otherwise. The causes can be classified by anatomical level along the urinary tract (ie originating from the kidney, ureter, bladder, prostate, urethra) and it is worth thinking about hameaturia in this way when eliciting the history.

Although this gentleman is on **anticoagulation** for AF, which may exacerbate his haematuria, it should not be presumed that this is the sole cause for his symptoms and based on the above statement ('cancer until proven otherwise'), other causes should be excluded first.

Indeed, this patient is presenting with two symptoms out of a classic triad of symptoms typically seen in **renal cell carcinoma** (macroscopic haematuria, renal mass and loin pain), although the classic triad only occurs in 10–15% cases.

Other causes to be considered are **prostate** pathology (prostate carcinoma, BPH), **UTIs**, urinary **calculi** and **glomerulonephritis**, although these are less likely given the above history.

➤ Case 12

You are a GP trainee. A 40-year-old woman has come to see you complaining of a painful right knee.

Please take a detailed history from her to determine the cause of the problem.

What questions would you like to ask the patient?

PC

One week history of red, hot, swollen and painful right knee.

HPC

Site – right knee only affected, no other joints.

Onset – came on quickly, persistent with no triggering factors.

Character – painful, red, swollen, hot.

Radiation – nil radiation.

Associated symptoms – ODQ stiffness of joint, intermittent low-grade fevers.

ODQ has had some recent rectal bleeding, loose stools and weight loss.

No eye, skin, urinary symptoms.

Timing - no real diurnal variation for pain and/or stiffness.

Exacerbating/ **R**elieving factors – NSAIDs make it slightly better but still quite severe.

No history of recent trauma.

PMHx

Fit and well. No significant past medical or surgical history.

DHx

NSAIDs for joint pain (ibuprofen PRN).

NKDA. No OTC medications.

SHx

Non-smoker.

Drinks 20 units alcohol a week.

No recent travel history.

FHx

ODQ father had ankylosing spondylitis.

SE

Nil

What is your differential diagnosis?

What investigations would you like to carry out?

Case discussion

Serious causes of monoarticular joint problems must be excluded first, namely **septic arthritis**. The knee is affected in more than half of all cases of septic arthritis.

Gout is another possibility given the weekly alcohol consumption. It is important to be aware that no other joint is involved so this makes **rheumatoid arthritis** less likely, although cannot be completely excluded until further investigations are undertaken. The acute history makes **osteoarthritis** less likely and symptoms are suggestive of an inflammatory aetiology as a cause for this patient's symptoms.

Systemic diseases, such as **SLE**, are less likely given that this is a monoarticular presentation.

It is important to pick up on the associated bowel symptoms in this case, along with the positive family history of ankylosing spondylitis. This raises the possibility of a **seronegative spondyloarthropathy** (HLA-B27-associated), such as **enteropathic arthritis**, which may cause an oligoarthritis with an asymmetrical presentation.

Initial investigations to determine a diagnosis would include blood tests, blood cultures, a knee aspiration and an X-ray.

➤ Case 13

You are a GP trainee doctor. An 82-year-old woman has come to see you complaining of a skin problem.

Please take a detailed history from her to determine the cause of the problem.

What questions would you like to ask the patient?

P C

Complaining of a crusty, slow growing skin ulcer on her left shin.

H P C

Site – left, anterior shin.

Onset – noticed 2 weeks ago following a traumatic episode, getting larger.

Character – ulcerated, not pigmented.

Radiation – no other lesions elsewhere.

Associated symptoms – no bleeding, some itching associated with lesion. Patient feels scratching it has caused it to get worse.

P MHx

Background of Bowen's disease.

Has ulcerative colitis.

D Hx

Azathioprine for inflammatory bowel disease.

Vitamin supplements.

Allergic to peanuts.

Has a holiday home in Spain and enjoys sunbathing.

Functionally independent.

Smokes 10 a day (since age 20).

Nil alcohol.

FHx

Nil of note.

SE

Nil.

What is your differential diagnosis?

What investigations would you like to carry out?

Case discussion

When considering patients with skin lesions, the serious malignant causes that require exclusion are **malignant melanoma**, **squamous cell carcinoma** and **basal cell carcinoma**. The predominant risk factor for all these skin tumours is sun exposure. The fact that this patient enjoys sunbathing in Spain, that the lesion is present in a sun-exposed area and is also ulcerated makes all of these conditions a distinct possibility in this lady.

This patient has several additional risk factors for squamous cell carcinoma, including a past history of Bowen's disease (a pre-malignant condition) and the presence of immunosuppression (azathioprine). This makes **squamous cell carcinoma** the most likely diagnosis. The history of the lesion following a traumatic episode is a 'red herring' in this case, but a **pyogenic granuloma, dermatofibroma** or a **traumatised seborrhoeic keratosis (seborrheoic wart)** could be considered.

Other benign conditions that also require exclusion are **keratoacanthoma** (which mimics a squamous cell carcinoma and grows rapidly) and a **solar (actinic) keratosis** (a pre-malignant condition).

A biopsy is warranted here to make a formal diagnosis.

➤ Case 14

You are the foundation year urologist on call. A 16-year-old boy has been referred to you by A&E complaining of testicular pain.

Please take a detailed history from him to determine the cause of the problem.

What questions would you like to ask the patient?

P C

Sudden onset pain, following a rugby match.

HPC

Site – left scrotum.

Onset – sudden onset 3–4 hours ago, which has got progressively worse following a rugby match.

Character – dull ache in scrotum.

Radiation – no radiation to groin, or elsewhere.

Associated symptoms – no urinary or bowel symptoms, no abdominal pain, no urethral discharge, skin not red/hot, testis feels 'swollen'.

Timing – progressively getting more painful.

Exacerbating factors – worse with walking.

Severity – too painful to touch.

PMHx

Not had any similar episodes, or infections (STIs).

Not noticed any scrotal lump/swellings preceding this incident.

History of left maldescended testis (cryptorchidism).

Otherwise fit and well.

DHx

Nil regular medications.

SHx

Sexually active – one partner.

Non-smoker.

Nil alcohol.

FHx

Nil of note.

SE

Nil

What is your differential diagnosis?

What investigations would you like to carry out?

Case discussion

It is of prime important to consider the most serious cause of scrotal pain, namely **testicular torsion**, in the first instance, especially given the history of trauma in this case. This patient will require further examination and investigations to exclude this diagnosis, which may necessitate an exploration in theatre. However, **incarcerated/strangulated inguinal hernias** are also important to consider.

A **haematocele** is important to think about in light of the trauma and one must never forget the possibility of a **testicular tumour** which likewise commonly presents with a history of trauma (where the trauma brings the tumour to the attention of the patient). A history of cryptorchidism (maldescended testis), as in this case, increases the risk of a testicular torsion, testicular tumours and subfertility.

As this gentleman is sexually active, **epididymo-orchitis** is also a possible diagnosis. Other differentials such as **varicocele**, **epididymal cyst** and **hydrocele** are unlikely given the acute history and severity of pain. Always consider referred pain such as **ureteric colic**.

Initial investigations to help determine the diagnosis would include blood tests, urine dipstick and microscopy, scrotal ultrasound scan and STI screening.

Index